Victorian
CSI

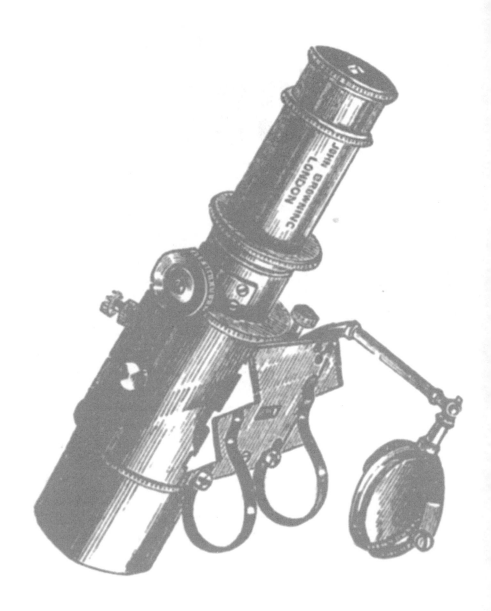

VICTORIAN
CSI

William A. Guy, David Ferrier & William R. Smith

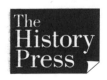

First published 1844
This edition 2009

The History Press
The Mill, Brimscombe Port
Stroud, Gloucestershire, GL5 2QG
www.thehistorypress.co.uk

British Library Cataloguing in Publication Data.
A catalogue record for this book is available from the British Library.

ISBN 978 0 7524 5513 6

Typesetting and origination by The History Press
Printed in Great Britain

Contents

PRINCIPLES

OF

FORENSIC MEDICINE.

INTRODUCTION.

THE State avails itself of the knowledge, experience, and skill of the medical man for three distinct purposes:—1. For the care of soldiers and sailors, prisoners, paupers, lunatics, and others for whose safety it makes itself responsible; 2. As officers of health and analysts; and 3. As skilled witnesses in courts of law.

The duties of the medical man in the first of these capacities are such as devolve upon him in the ordinary practice of his profession; but he is expected to prevent as well as to cure disease, and to add to professional skill administrative ability.

As medical officers of health, however, and as witnesses in courts of law, medical men have duties to perform for which the ordinary practice of their profession affords no adequate preparation; medical education, till of late years, no proper training; and medical literature no sufficient guidance.

The distinctness, importance, and difficulty of these duties led at length to the establishment of a distinct science, taught in separate courses of lectures, treated in separate works, and engaging the attention of men more or less separated and set apart for the practice of the corresponding art.

This new science either embraced all the duties the medical man may be required to perform on behalf of the State, in which case it received the name of Political or State Medicine; or it was divided into two sciences, the one known as Hygiene or Public Health, the other as Forensic Medicine, Juridical Medicine, Legal Medicine, or Medical Jurisprudence.

As regards the second of these, the term Forensic Medicine expresses with sufficient clearness the application of medical knowledge to legal purposes, and consequently it is used in the title of this work. The term medico-legal is also in common use, as in the phrases " medico-legal knowledge," "medico-legal experience," " medico-legal skill."

It is to be regretted that this division of State Medicine has not made the same progress in this country as that of Hygiene or Public Health, a fact doubtless due to the difficulty of obtaining practical experience by those who are teachers of the subject.

In reference to the first of these sciences, Hygiene or Public Health, it is no part of our present duty to deal, but be it noted that in this department of State Medicine a registrable qualification is now obtainable only after compliance with a strict curriculum of study, and the possession of such qualification is necessary for all the more important Public Health appointments.

The history of Forensic Medicine is that of most other sciences. Necessity or convenience gives birth to an art practised by persons more or less skilful, without guidance from general principles ; but its importance, and the responsibility attached to the practice of it, soon create a demand for instruction, oral and written, which gradually assumes a systematic form. Thus it was that the Science of Medicine sprang from an empirical art of healing. In like manner, the Science of Forensic Medicine took its rise in the necessity of bringing medical knowledge to bear on legal inquiries relating to injuries or loss of life ; the medical witness being at first without guidance in the performance of his duty, and so continuing till a growing sense of the important bearing of his work on the interests of society, and on his own reputation, created a demand for instruction that could not fail of being supplied. Cases were accordingly collected, arranged, and commented on, illustrative facts sought after, special experiments devised and performed, till at length the medical witness received in books and lectures the same distinct instruction as the physician or surgeon at the bedside had already derived from written or oral teaching in the theory and practice of medicine, or of surgery.

But the importance of medical testimony received an earlier recognition from Continental Governments than from the public or the medical profession ; for the first State recognition (1507) anticipated by nearly a century the first medico-legal treatise

(1597); and the first appointment of medical men to perform medico-legal duties followed soon after, in France, in 1603.*

The history of Forensic Medicine in England is of more recent date. It begins with the publication, in 1788, of Dr. Samuel Farr's "Elements of Medical Jurisprudence," and the subject was first taught in lectures at Edinburgh, in 1801, by Dr. Duncan. sen., the first professorship being conferred by Government on his son in the University of that city in 1803. In England the first professorship was created in King's College, London, Sir Thomas Watson being appointed to the chair in 1831. The new science soon justified the distinction thus conferred upon it, and made good its claims to more general recognition. It is now taught in all our medical schools, and recognised by the examining bodies; its principles are being constantly applied in our courts of law; and England continues to contribute her fair share of observation and research towards its extension and improvement.

The application of the principles of the science—in other words, the practice of it as an art—devolves, for the most part, on the medical practitioner. But those specially versed in the entire subject, or in important parts of it (such as Toxicology), or eminent in certain branches of practice (such as midwifery and the treatment of the insane), are occasionally summoned to give evidence.

There are many reasons why the medical man should approach this class of duties with apprehension. He is conscious of the importance that attaches to his evidence; he is wanting in the confidence which a more frequent appearance as a witness would impart; he is painfully alive to the unstable foundation on which many medical opinions rest; he knows that it is not easy in practice to observe the rules of evidence with which in theory he may have made himself acquainted; and, above all, he shrinks from the publicity attendant on legal proceedings, the unreason-

---

* The following dates have an historic interest :—The penal code of the Bishop of Bamberg, proclaimed 1507. A uniform penal code adopted by the Diet of Ratisbon, 1532. "Constitutio Criminalis Caroline," published 1553. Letters patent, presented to his first physician by Henry IV. of France, empowering him to appoint two surgeons in every city and large town to examine and report on wounded or murdered persons, 1603. Publication at Frankfort of the Methodus Testificandi of Condronchus, 1597, and of the works of Fortunatus Fidelis and Paul Zacchias in 1598 and 1621. First course of lectures on Forensic Medicine by Michaelis at Leipzig about 1650. See Traill's "Outlines of Medical Jurisprudence.

able licence allowed to counsel, and the disparaging comments of the Bench itself.

Sympathising in these reasonable apprehensions, some writers of eminence, and most authors on Forensic Medicine, have tried to prepare the medical witness for his duties by setting forth in more or less detail the precautions he should observe both prior to and during his attendance in court ; and by special directions for conducting medico-legal inquiries under the heads of " Post-mortem inspection," " General evidence of poisoning," " Unsoundness of mind," etc. ; the general precautions to be observed in the witness-box being made the subject of distinct treatment under the title Medical Evidence.

Before treating of the duties of the medical witness, it may be well to show the number of cases that occur year by year in England and Wales of a class to give rise to medico-legal inquiries. The following figures are extracted from the Annual Report of the Registrar-General for the year 1892 :—

Deaths by accident or negligence, suicide, murder,
    and manslaughter   19,226
Premature births, congenital malformations, and
    atelectasis   20,019
Ill-defined and non-specified causes .   .   . 25,176

Total . 64,421

The following special causes of death were recorded in the year 1892 :—

Causes of Death.	Accident or Neglect.	Suicide	Total.	Males.	Females.
Poison	514	301	815	517	298
Fractures and bruises . . .	6,769	152	6,921	5,342	1,579
Gunshot	102	261	363	352	11
Cuts and stabs	29	501	530	413	117
Burns and scalds	2,369	8	2,377	1,074	1,303
Drowning	2,637	584	3221	2,574	647
Hanging	...	671	671	532	139
Suffocation	2,166	...	2,166	1,180	986
Otherwise	1,757	105	1,862	1,309	553
Total	16,343	2,583	18,926	13,293	5,633

In the same year (1892), the deaths by accident or negligence were distributed between the sexes as follows :—Poison, men 340, women 174; Gunshot, men 95, women 7; Cuts and stabs, men 20, women 9; Drowning, men 2231, women 406; otherwise, men 1222, women 535.

The suicides were distributed as follows:—Poison, men 177, women 124; Gunshot, men 257, women 4; Cuts and stabs, men 393, women 108; Drowning, men 343, women 241; Hanging, men 532, women 139; otherwise, men 87, women 18.

In the year 1892 the premature, sudden, and violent deaths gave rise to 32,254 inquests, and as the qualified practitioners in England and Wales fall far short of this number, it follows that, if medical evidence were called for at every inquest, and the duty of attending at inquests were distributed equally, each member of the profession would attend at least one inquest every year.

The committals for trial arising out of these 32,254 inquests amounted to 180, of which 76 were for murder and 104 for manslaughter. In 2545 instances the death was returned as suicidal.

The number of cases requiring medical evidence in our higher courts of law may be judged of approximately from the printed returns of commitments for trial for offences against the person. In the year 1891-2 these amounted to 1859, and comprised—

Murder and attempts to murder	138
Various attempts to maim and injure . . .	425
Assaults	256
Manslaughter	104
Concealment of birth	36
Rape and assaults with intent	499
Unnatural offences	97
	1555[*]

If we add to the occasions for medical evidence arising out of these crimes, the civil cases in which skilled medical evidence is required, and proceedings in respect of lunatics, the occasions on which medical men are summoned to courts of law, either in the service of the State or on behalf of individuals, will appear very considerable—certainly numerous enough, and important enough in themselves, to justify all the attempts which have been made to construct a science of Forensic Medicine, to teach it systematic-

[*] These figures are taken from the annual report, entitled "Judicial Statistics" (England and Wales), 1892.

ally in books and lectures, and to draw up a code of instructions for the guidance of the medical witness in the performance of his duties.

MEDICAL EVIDENCE.

The medical man may, like any other person, be summoned as a witness merely to state facts which have come within his knowledge, in which case he will occupy the position of an ordinary or common witness; or he may be called to express an opinion upon facts observed by him as a medical man at the request of friends or others, or upon the views held by other skilled observers in reference to such facts; in each of these cases he becomes a skilled or expert witness.

In performing these duties there are certain precautions which the witness ought to observe, and certain legal requirements of which he should not be ignorant.

1. He should " use his best endeavours that his mind be clear and collected, unawed by fear, and uninfluenced by favour or enmity." (Percival.) He will not find it easy to maintain this impartial frame of mind when the crime alleged is one of unusual enormity; when popular feeling runs high for or against the accused; or, in times of public agitation, when his evidence tends to discredit some popular movement or deep-rooted prejudice. Nor, when he is engaged as a skilled witness, or *expert*, for the prosecution or for the defence, must he deem himself free from the risk of partiality, even though, after hearing all the facts which should influence his opinion, he feels that he can conscientiously give his evidence in support of the side for which he is retained.

2. The medical witness requires to be specially cautioned against expressing an opinion on the general merits of the case under inquiry, thus offending against an admitted principle of English law, that "when scientific men are called as witnesses, they are not entitled to give their opinion as to the merits of the case, but only as to the facts proved on the trial.

3. A special caution is also required against indulging a feeling of misplaced humanity, or an equally misplaced condemnation of the law on the score of undue severity. Both these feelings too often found expression in former treatises on the lung-tests and in early trials for infanticide. But the witness should understand

that he is not responsible for the consequences to which his opinions may lead, provided always that they are the result of cautious inquiry and due reflection. Percival accordingly treats "the dread of innocent blood being brought upon us by explicit and honest testimony," as "one of those superstitions which the nurse has taught, and which a liberal education ought to purge from the mind."

The witness approaching his duties with a mind thus free from bias, requires some instruction as to the mode in which his evidence should be given.

1. Bearing in mind the distinction just laid down between a common and a skilled witness, he should be cautious not to obtrude his opinions when facts only are required of him, nor dogmatically to assert as facts things which are merely matters of opinion. He should answer the questions put to him, whether by counsel, court, or jury, clearly and concisely, and if these do not elicit the whole truth, it is quite competent for him to offer to the court such explanation as he may think necessary.

2. His statements should be made, and his opinions expressed, in the plainest and simplest language; and he should avoid as much as possible all technical terms, and all figurative and metaphorical expressions—e.g., a blood clot is a better witness-box expression than an apoplectic extravasation, and a bruise is a phrase better understood than a contusion.

3. The medical witness ought also to abstain from quoting authorities in support of his opinions; for though the rule of exclusion has not always been rigidly acted on, the common usage of our courts of law is certainly to disallow these appeals. Nor is this exclusion open to any serious objection, for the witness is supposed to make himself master of the views of the most eminent writers on the subject matter of his evidence, and to use them as aids and guides to his own special inquiries.

But though the witness may not cite authorities, he may be asked whether A. or B. is an esteemed authority with his profession, and whether he (the witness) coincides with some opinion expressed in his works. If the witness answers in the affirmative, he becomes the exponent of the opinion to which he thus gives his assent. The medical witness should carefully avoid all flippancy of manner and exaggerations in language, and give his evidence in a concise, plain, and clear manner.

The foregoing observations relate chiefly to the mode in which the witness should give his evidence. The precautions to be observed in order that his evidence may be admissible still remain to be considered, under the following heads :—

1. **Notes.**—When observing any facts which, at a future time, may become the subject-matter for legal inquiry, the medical man should not trust to his memory, but commit them to writing, either on the spot, or as soon as possible after the transaction to which they relate. If (as in performing a post-mortem examination) it is necessary to resort to dictation, the notes of the amanuensis should be immediately examined and corrected.

The witness may use these notes in court to refresh his memory, but not to supply its place. If they were not made till some time after the events to which they refer, or if, having been made at the proper time, they have been entirely forgotten, they will not be admissible.

2. **Confessions.**—A culprit may make a confession of guilt to his medical attendant. This, to be admissible in a court of law, must be free and voluntary, uninfluenced by threat, promise, or bribe. No sort of inducement should be held out to make it, no leading questions should be put, and no comments made; but the medical man should reduce the statement to writing as soon as possible, read it over to the person confessing, obtain his signature to it, and countersign it himself.

At the same time the greatest care should be taken to ascertain the bodily health and mental state of the party making the confession. The necessity of this caution has been amply proved by cases in which, during febrile attacks, or after prolonged exposure and hardship, as well as in cases of delusional insanity, confessions have been made of murders and other heinous crimes which had never been committed. In times now happily passed away, innocent persons, under like conditions of body and mind, made confession of impossible crimes, such as witchcraft.

3. **Death-bed or Dying Declarations.**—These are admitted as evidence in cases of homicide, where the death of the deceased is the subject of the charge, and the circumstances of the fatal injury the subject of the declaration. It is assumed that the declarant having lost all hope of recovery, is induced to speak the truth by considerations as powerful as an oath administered in a court of justice. It is not necessary, however, that he should

express his conviction. It may be inferred from the nature of the injury, or from other circumstances of the case. But if any hope whatever be entertained, or may be inferred to exist, whether it be spontaneous or on the suggestion of others, death-bed declarations cannot be received in evidence.* The case of Reg. *v.* Mitchell, March 22, 1892 (Mr. Justice Cave, Nottingham Assizes), is interesting as showing how strict the law is in reference to the admission of dying declarations. The prisoner was indicted for the murder of a woman by procuring a miscarriage by the use of instruments or other means, death resulting therefrom. It was held that upon an indictment for murder or manslaughter, a statement giving the substance of questions put to, and answers given by, the deceased person is not admissible in evidence as a dying declaration; such a declaration to be admissible must be in the actual words of the deceased, and if questions be put, both the questions and answers must be given, in order to show how much was suggested by the questioner and how much answered by the deceased. In this case the deceased was told by the medical attendant there was little or no hope for her, and when asked if she understood her position, replied that she did. It was held, there was no proof of a settled or hopeless expectation of immediate death sufficient to make a subsequent declaration admissible as a dying declaration, and although the deceased said she understood what the doctor said, there was nothing to show that she agreed with him.

But the person, or persons, inculpated by the declarant's statement are not precluded from giving evidence as to his state of mind and behaviour in his last moments. They may be allowed to show that the deceased was influenced by vindictive motives, or was not of a character to be " impressed by a religious sense of his approaching dissolution."

As dying declarations are but confessions of the most solemn kind, the same rules of procedure apply to them as to confessions.

---

* In a case (Trial of Bedingfield for the murder of Mrs. Rudd, Nov. 1879) Lord Chief Justice Cockburn, by not treating as a dying declaration what other high legal authorities would have considered as a part of the *res gestæ*, and therefore admissible, shut out an important piece of evidence. " A woman's scream was heard from the house, and immediately afterwards the deceased was seen coming out with her throat cut, making a statement which, according to the rules of evidence, was not admissible, and in about ten minutes she was dead." Mr. Pitt-Taylor, in a letter to the *Times* (Nov. 15, 1879), quotes no less than five legal authorities in favour of his opinion that the statement of the woman Rudd ought to have been admitted as part of the *res gestæ.*

The medical man should put no leading questions, but only such as are necessary to clear up ambiguity. He should commit the declaration to writing, read it to the dying man, and obtain his assent, and, if possible, his signature to it. But if this cannot be done, he should make a memorandum of the declaration at once, while it and the words used are fresh in his memory. To this document the witness will be allowed to refer, to refresh his memory, when he comes to give evidence. Another essential part of his duty is to ascertain the exact state of the declarant's mind, whether he is calm and collected, or otherwise, and whether he is under the influence of any strong bias or undue feeling of resentment.

4. **Hearsay**.—This is not admissible as evidence unless it form part of the *res gestæ*. A medical witness, therefore, though he may state in evidence the words he has heard used in direct reference to the case which forms the subject of inquiry, could not cite a case in support of his opinions if it consisted in part, as it must needs do, of statements made by the patient, his friends, or attendants.

5. **Secrets**.—The medical man, in the course of his professional attendance, may receive secret information which under ordinary circumstances he would be bound not to divulge. But it should be understood that in a court of justice he may be compelled to divulge these secrets.

It is now no longer necessary to warn the medical man against taking part in duels, even though his object in being present is to save life, and not to destroy it. But if in this, or in any other way, he has acted illegally, he, in common with other witnesses, is not obliged to criminate himself.

6. **Wills**.—A medical man may be required, on an emergency, to draft the will of a patient, or to witness the instrument. In taking the instructions of the testator, he should limit himself to such inquiries as may enable him to understand his wishes. He should write them in the fewest, simplest, and clearest words on one side of a sheet of paper, append the place and exact date of the transaction, and at the foot of the document (leaving room for two signatures) the following words :—"Signed by the above-named testator, in the presence of us present at the same time, who have hereunto signed our names as witnesses thereto, in the presence of the said testator, and in presence of each other." The

testator and witnesses must attach their signatures in accordance with these words, for the validity of the will depends in the main upon them. Witnesses to a will cannot be beneficiaries under the will.

The medical man should take care to observe the condition, bodily and mental, of the testator ; and he would do well to make a note of all the circumstances of the case while they are fresh in his memory. Wills so made have been disputed, and the medical man has been summoned as a witness, and submitted to a searching examination.

PART I.

CHAPTER I.

PERSONAL IDENTITY. AGE. SEX.

WHEN called upon to examine the body or remains of some unknown person, we may have first to ascertain the sex and the age, and then to identify the individual by characteristic marks; or these points may have to be considered separately, both in living and in dead persons. The three subjects are here grouped together, and placed in the most convenient order; sex last, from its connection with the subjects of Chapter II.

PERSONAL IDENTITY.

Questions of identity are often raised in courts of law; as when a claim is set up to an inheritance, or a man who has been robbed or assaulted has to identify the thief or the person who has injured him. A witness may also be required to identify an acquaintance; and a jury may be empanelled for the sole purpose of trying the question of the identity of an escaped prisoner. So also as to persons found dead; and in coroners' inquests the first step taken is to identify the body, or such parts of it as are forthcoming.

The subject of personal identity, then, divides itself into—

I. THE IDENTITY OF THE LIVING. II. THE IDENTITY OF THE DEAD.

I. IDENTITY OF THE LIVING.

The medical man may be required to examine, with a view to identification, alleged deformities or injuries, scars, or discolorations of the skin or hair; and to express an opinion on the changes that may be wrought in stature, face, and person by time, exposure, and hardship. It is also within his province to give evidence on the influence of the like causes on the mind and memory.

In order to give completeness to this subject, some questions will be briefly noticed in which medical evidence is not needed.

In cases of disputed inheritance much stress is laid on family resemblance. The celebrated Douglas Peerage case was decided in favour of the claimant, Archibald Douglas, in consequence of his proved resemblance to Colonel Stewart, his father; the twin brother, Sholto, who died young, having equally resembled Mrs. Stewart, the mother. In this case, Lord Mansfield strongly insisted on this resemblance of child to parent, as well as on the strongly contrasted fact that, in an army one hundred thousand strong, every man may be known from another; if not by feature, size, attitude, and action, by voice, gestures, smile, and expression.

Though these statements generally hold good (and not of men only, but of herds of cattle and flocks of sheep), still there are not wanting instances of persons having no connection by relationship or descent who have yet borne the closest resemblance to each other. Of this mistaken identity, Lord Chief Justice Cockburn, in the Tichborne case, cited, among other illustrations, a case on the Western Circuit, in which two men were tried and convicted for murder. The identity of one of them was sworn to by numerous witnesses; but it was afterwards proved that at the very time of the murder he was undergoing punishment for picking a pocket hundreds of miles away. A most curious case of this kind occurred in 1772, when one Mall, a barber's apprentice, was tried at the Old Bailey for robbing a Mrs. Ryan. The witnesses swore to his identity, and the whole court thought him guilty; but on referring to the books of the court it appeared that on the day and hour of the robbery he was on his trial at the bar where he then stood for another robbery, in which he was likewise mistaken for the thief.

When the question of identity turns on the changes which time, coupled perhaps with fatigues, hardships. and privations, may work in the personal appearance, it becomes one of unusual difficulty. Cassali, a noble Bolognese, left his country at an early age, and was supposed to have died in battle; but, after thirty years, returned and claimed his property, which his heirs had appropriated. His appearance was so changed that he was imprisoned as an impostor. Zacchias was consulted, and, in his report, expressed his opinion that such a change might have been wrought by age, change of climate, diet, mode of life, and disease, and as Cassali had left home in the bloom of youth, had been exposed to the hardships of a military life, and, if he might be believed, had languished for years in prison, the judges, influenced by this opinion, and by the fact that the heirs could not prove the death of Cassali, decreed the restoration of his estates.

The general question thus submitted to Zacchias assumes a more definite form when, as in the French cases of Baronet and Martin Guerre, a false claimant is confronted with a real one, or alleges his identity with a person long since dead, as in the Tichborne case,* or when, as in this case, the claimant is alleged not only not to be the man he is personating, but some other person.

In all such cases of disputed identity great importance attaches to the existence, or absence, of such marks as nævi, moles, deformities, scars of previous disease or injury, and tattoo markings. The Tichborne case has also given renewed importance to the effect of lapse of time in changing the stature, form, and features, and in destroying or modifying the memory and habits of thought, as expressed in words spoken or written; and it has shown the importance that may attach to photographs, as the most exact representation possible of the personal appearance at the time when they were taken.

Scars and Tattoo Markings.—1. **Scars.**—When a claimant presents himself without the marks or scars known to have characterised the individual whom he personates, his case must break down under personal examination; but if these marks or scars are found upon him, they are the strongest possible evidence in his favour, and would, indeed, be conclusive but that they may have been fraudulently imitated, or they may be coincidences which although improbable are not impossible. That such coincidences may happen, is proved by the case, quoted by Beck, of Joseph

---

* The reader will find the cases of Cassali, Baronet, and Martin Guerre, with the other leading cases from the "Causes Célèbres," quoted and criticised by Foderé in the second chapter of his "Traité de Médecine Légale"; and he is referred for a lucid account of the extraordinary case of Martin Guerre to the *Times*, December 12, 1871. It is the case in which Arnauld de Tilh, who had possessed himself of the secrets of Martin, contrived to be recognised by his family, and even accepted, seemingly in good faith, by Martin's wife. (See a brief abstract of this case appended to this chapter.)

Parker, tried at New York in 1804, for bigamy. He was mistaken for Thomas Hoag, whom he not merely resembled, but had in common with him a scar on the forehead, a small mark on the neck, and a lisp in his speech; but, unlike Hoag, no scar on the foot. That he was Parker, and not Hoag, was proved to the satisfaction of the jury by an alibi.

Removal and disappearance of scars.—The question of identity has sometimes turned on the possibility of removing scars, upon which some difference of opinion has been expressed. Thus, in a Belgian case that occurred in 1847, M. Vandelaer stated that scars might be removed by time or by artificial means, and the physicians of the prisons of Valvorde and Ghent confirmed this opinion by stating that prisoners are in the habit of effacing scars by applying a salted herring to them. MM. Lebeau and Limanges, on the other hand, contended that scars could not be removed. On this subject Casper states that the length of time during which a scar subsists depends on the depth to which the tissues of the skin have been injured. Scars of superficial injuries which have only affected the epidermis, or scarf skin, and left the true skin intact, may entirely disappear. But we may confidently assert that even the slight wounds caused by bleeding or cupping, if they have penetrated the whole depth of the cutaneous tissues, and, *à fortiori*, such wounds, injuries, or ulcers as have caused loss of substance, followed by granulation, leave behind them permanent scars.

Scars may, however, fade with the lapse of time; and, on the other hand, owing to their slight vascularity as compared with the surrounding skin, be rendered more distinct by friction, pressure, blows, or irritants. Thus, Devergie states that the white brand-mark of the galley-slave which has apparently disappeared may be rendered visible by slapping the spot with the hand till it reddens.

The belief that the effects of injuries may wholly disappear is probably founded on the very slight marks left by extensive wounds when they heal by what is technically called the "first intention." Thus, in the case of a maniac who had completely removed the parts of generation, the place of the wound was marked by a faint white line, which a casual observer might overlook; and the severe floggings of former times, which left the back quite raw, are traceable after some years only by fine white lines on the back and sides, and, where the knots had fallen, by little circular pits. In a case in which we were consulted, the entire absence of both kinds of mark enabled us to state with confidence that the man could not have been, as was alleged, very severely flogged (G.).*

The removal of scars has another important bearing on the question of identification. It may happen that an impostor, aware that evidence will be forthcoming that he has certain tattoo or other superficial marks on his person which the man he is personating had not, resorts to heat or strong corrosives, or such agents as the vaccine virus, to erase the marks in question. The substituted marks thus become a very strong presumption of imposition, especially if the person bearing these marks cannot or will not explain the way in which they were produced, or offers some explanation that refutes itself. It will be presently shown that the claimant in the Tichborne case had two such marks on his left arm.

Shape, situation, and depth of scars.—The cause of a scar may often be inferred from its appearance, and the situation in which it is found. Thus, a linear scar, or a round or oval surface scar, on the arm, ankle, or temple, follows bleeding; parallel linear scars on the loins, shoulders, nape of neck, or other fleshy part, would be the result of cupping; a crucial linear scar on any part of the body would indicate a boil treated by incision; two parallel linear scars on the nape of the neck, shoulder, or inner side of the upper arm, would mark a seton; and a depressed, puckered scar on the same parts, an issue; a honeycombed disc near the insertion of the deltoid muscle indicates the operation of vaccination; a white disc with dotted border may follow a boil that has healed without operation; and every form of cicatrix in the neck, on the chest, and elsewhere may follow scrofulous abscesses. Scrofula, small-pox, syphilis, and lupus, in common with injuries by gunshot, burns, and escharotics, may leave behind them scars of every size and form.

Changes in colour of scars.—All scars, without exception, pass through two distinct stages—that of inflammatory redness (the immediate consequence of the injury sustained) and that of

---

* Of the permanency of such scars as those left by bleeding, a good illustration is afforded by a case in which two physicians, one 66, and the other 64 years of age, having distinct recollection that they were bled in the arm at about 7 years, and not since, the marks of the operation were in both cases perfectly distinct (G.).

brown discoloration. In phlegmonous erysipelas, and after the application of blisters, mustard poultices, and other strong irritants, the skin, which was red during the inflammatory stage, assumes a dark brown or coppery hue. This it retains for months, and even for three or four years. At length, and by degrees, the skin resumes its healthy colour. But sometimes, when the inflammation runs high, the brown discoloration is followed by a third stage, or that of bleaching. Thus we have seen, after the lapse of two years and a half, the spot to which a large blister had been applied defined by a white margin, and white decoloration occupying the whole surface on a level with the surrounding healthy skin (G. 1. Such *surface scars* follow the less severe forms of herpes, boils that heal after slight destruction of texture, and even incised wounds and lancet cuts, where the edges have not been brought together, and some slight superficial ulceration has taken place. In those cases in which the inflammation, however produced, is followed by ulceration, and consequent destruction of tissue, and still more where gangrene sets in, the scars are wholly or in part sunk beneath the surface. In these cases, too, the scar passes through the three stages of inflammatory redness, brown discoloration, and bleaching.

The cicatricial tissue is wanting in the characteristics of true skin; it has neither sebaceous nor sweat glands and no hair follicles.

Healing of scars.—This is influenced by many causes, such as age, constitution, and state of health, the situation of the scar on flat, rounded, or hollow surfaces, on parts subject or not subject to motion, and in the direction of muscles or across them.

Distinctness of Scars.—This will depend on the complexion, and the tint of parts adjacent. Thus, scars are less apparent in persons of fair complexion, when the skin approaches in tint to the whiteness of the scar itself, and more distinct over a blue vein or discoloured portion of skin.

Age of Scars.—As has been stated, all scars, whether arising from injury or disease, are first red, then brown, then white and glistening. The redness, as a rule, lasts two, three, or four weeks, during the period of healing; the brown discoloration for several months, or even for a few years; the bleached appearance for the rest of life. But the duration of each stage is subject to great variation, as is seen in some cases of small-pox, where the scars are white and shining at the end of six months, while in others they remain brown even after two or three years. Scrofulous ulcers, too, sometimes leave coloured scars for the whole of life. A scar, then, that retains its inflammatory redness cannot be of long standing; one that has a brown or coppery colour may have existed for months or years; a white glistening scar, quite free from colour, must have been of long standing; but we cannot even guess at its age.

Some scars are parti-coloured, perhaps brown in the central parts, with a white puckered halo; or white in the centre with a brown margin. Thus a scar of ten years' standing from a boil consisted of a white disc, with a circular margin of brown spots. Sometimes we have an opportunity of comparing a recent scar with one of longer standing due to the same cause, as in a prisoner who had two attacks of herpes, one under the right, the other under the left clavicle. The first, of a few months' standing, displayed the rash in all its details in dark brown; the second, of many years' standing, consisted of a group of scattered white cicatrices. Scars made during infancy increase in size with the growth of the body.

Rules for examining scars.—Place the scar, if possible, in the bright light of the sun, and, in the case of small and delicate scars, use a lens. Measure the scar carefully with compasses, and note its exact dimensions. Record the form and colour of the several parts of which it consists. Redden the surrounding skin by blows or friction. Note whether it is on a level with, or sunk beneath, the surrounding surface; and whether it moves with the skin or remains fixed.

2. **Tattoo markings.**—The presence or absence of these marks may, as in the Tichborne case, prove of the first importance; and the question naturally arises, whether these marks can disappear or be removed. Most tattoo marks are certainly indelible if not interfered with; but that they may in some cases disappear is proved by the observations of Casper, Hutin, and Tardieu; though these authorities differ widely as to the proportion of cases, Casper alleging the high fraction of 1 in 9, Tardieu the much lower one of 1 in 25. Much depends on the kind of colouring matter employed. Cinnabar, blue ink, and common ink create less permanent marks than Indian ink, soot, washing blue, coal-dust, or gunpowder. Skilfully performed tatooing with gunpowder may be pronounced indelible. The difference in the durability of the marks depends

on the relative solubility and chemical stability of the colouring matters. When they disappear, the colouring matter is found deposited in the nearest absorbent glands, where it may be found after death. The absorption of the colouring matter is rarely so complete as not to leave some traces behind.

Tattoo markings may be removed artificially; but if the pigment be deep in the skin, a cicatrix will be left in the spot where the marks existed. An experiment was made by Tardieu on a prisoner who had a crucifix tattooed with Indian ink on his forearm. After several applications of acetic acid, potash, and hydrochloric acid, a crust fell off at the end of fourteen days, leaving only a flat scar, without a trace of the original design. Escharotics will, of course, cause the disappearance of tattoo marks; but their place will be indicated by a permanent scar, sunk more or less below the level of the skin. The claimant in the Tichborne case had such a scar above the left wrist; and he had a very peculiar one on the left shoulder, which several insertions of vaccine matter at points equi-distant would be likely to produce. This scar occupied the place of the issue of three years' standing which Roger Tichborne had on the left shoulder; and it is therefore probable that it was intended to represent it.

Of tattoo marks, then, we may say that most of them are indelible; some disappear partially; a few entirely; and that if, in a dead body, these marks have disappeared, the colouring matter may be found in the nearest lymphatic glands.

Identification by photographs.—Photographs may mislead when used to represent the whole figure, inasmuch as the limbs, hands, and feet are not all in focus. But they may render great service when we are dealing with the fixed features of the face though the expression is less to be relied upon, for it is not quite the same in any two photographs taken by the same artist. Even these may vary according as they are in light or in shadow. In the Tichborne case photographs of Roger Tichborne, of the Claimant, and of members of the Orton family were all used at the trial, and served to show that the Claimant's face differed widely from that of Roger Tichborne taken twenty years before, and also that the Claimant bore a nearer resemblance to members of the Orton family than to Roger.[*]

* The illustrations in Figs. 1, 2, and 3 were executed under the direction of Mr. Piercy, the portrait painter, author of "A Crucial Test in Cases of Disputed Identity," with illustrations, 1873.

We will indicate some of the obvious uses of photographs.

1. **The eyes.**—The colour of the eyes and the direction of the line which joins the inner to the outer canthus, as well as the relative position and shape of the brows, are correctly indicated by photographs. Light blue and grey eyes print light, and hazel and brown eyes have a darker tint. By lines drawn through the inner and outer angles of the eyes and made to meet in the median line, we can determine whether the eyes have an upward or downward direction. All these points are well illustrated by the photographs produced in the Tichborne case. The iris in the upper of the two figures (Fig. 1), by its light tint, confirms the evidence of the

FIG. 1.

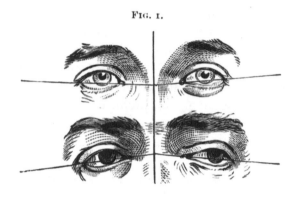

witnesses that the eyes of Roger were blue, while that of the lower figure, by its uniform dark colour, corresponds with the dark slate colour of the eye of the Claimant. In this same figure the lines drawn through the corners of the eyes indicate by their upward and downward direction a very important difference between the two persons. The photographs also show marked differences in the eyebrows. Those of Roger Tichborne are wide apart and singularly well defined, while those of the Claimant are much nearer together and of ill-defined outline.

2. **The ears.**—There are certain peculiarities in the ear, which may be deemed decisive. One of them consists in the absence of a pendulous lobe, and the firm adhesion of the point to the angle of the jaw; a second, in smallness or largeness of size; a third, in its direction relatively to the profile of the face; a fourth, in the rounded or angular outline, and the relative size and shape of its component parts. With the exception of the lobe of the ear, none of these peculiarities admit of being changed by any manipulation,

such as the use of weights or tension, and it is well known that that part is not greatly altered as the body grows and fattens. If artificial means were used to lengthen the lobe, they could not fail to be detected. The differences between the ears of Roger and the Claimant afford evidence which it is no exaggeration to term "startling." The ear of the Claimant is longer by one-third, the greater length being largely due to the detached pendulous lobe, which in Roger Tichborne did not exist. The dotted lines make the difference between the two ears very apparent Judging

by the published photographs, the ear of the Claimant closely resembles in size and shape that of George Orton, senior, and in size that of George Orton, junior.

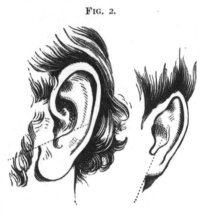

FIG. 2.

3. **The nose and mouth.—** These features, taken separately and together, admit of very marked contrasts. This fact, too, is well illustrated by the photographs produced in the Tichborne case. The nose of the Claimant, with which the lips may be said to harmonise, is "a narrow one in a fat face ;" that of Roger "a broad one, with inflated nostrils, in a thin face." The central groove which joins the nose to the upper lip, is narrow in the

FIG. 3.

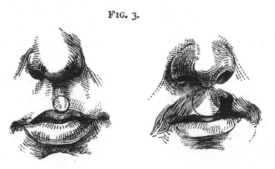

Claimant, wide in Roger—a difference well shown by the dotted circles in the figures. The two mouths are also quite different in character. The comparison, then, which these photographs enable us to institute between the face of Roger and that of the Claimant leaves no possible room for doubt that the actual personal appearance of the Claimant is not such as Roger Tichborne could have presented after the lapse of twenty years.

Identification by stature and girth.—In the Tichborne case these points came into play. Arthur Orton's Register Ticket, issued when he was 18, shows that he was 5 feet 9½ inches in his shoes, or 5 feet 9 inches in his stockings. The Claimant, carefully measured in his stockings in prison, was also 5 feet 9 inches. If, then, Arthur Orton stopped growing at 18, he and the Claimant might be one and the same person. But as men, one with another, grow two inches by the time they reach 30, there is a strong probability in favour of Orton having grown taller, and therefore against the Claimant and Orton being one and the same. In the case of Roger Tichborne, the Carabineer, the stature and girth of the chest were also put in evidence.

Identification by wounds.—In January 1846, when freshly-fallen snow was on the ground, a robbery was committed at Stigny, in the house of two old men. Next morning several spots of blood were seen on the floor on the left of a chest of drawers which the robbers had forced. Other spots were found on the snow in the direction taken by the robbers when they quitted the house, and always on the left hand of the footsteps. A shred of membrane was found on the road, which proved to be skin. On searching the neighbourhood, a man was found with his *left* hand wounded. Dr. Lemoine and M. Cœurderoi were appointed to examine him; and they agreed that the wound was probably inflicted about the date of the robbery, and that the piece of skin, judging from its size and shape, had formerly covered the injured part. The accused confessed the crime. ("Annales d'Hygiène," Jan. 1847.)

Alteration in the colour of the hair.—The question whether hair can be turned from dark to light was raised in Paris in 1832, on the occasion of the trial of one Bénoit for murder. Certain witnesses deposed to having seen him in Paris at 2 P.M. with black hair; while others declared that they saw him at Versailles, at 5 or 6 o'clock the same evening, with fair hair. The colour of the man's hair was jet black, and it does not appear that he wore a wig. The tribunal consulted Orfila, and Michalon, a leading hairdresser of Paris, as to the possibility of changing the hair from dark to light. Michalon replied in the negative; but Orfila stated that as early as the year 1806 Vauquelin had read at the Institute a *mémoire* on the property chlorine has of giving to black hair all the lighter colours, and even of bleaching it.

This case led to careful experiments by Orfila, and subsequently by Devergie. Orfila examined the mode of turning the hair from light to dark, from dark to light, and from light-red or chestnut to other shades of colour. Devergie limited himself to the verification of Orfila's experiments on the effect of chlorine.

Change from dark to light. — The results of numerous experiments made by Orfila and Devergie with solutions of chlorine may be thus summed up. Black hair is changed to various shades of chestnut, blond, yellow, and yellowish-white, by being steeped or washed, a longer or shorter time, in solutions of chlorine of different strengths. Less marked effects are produced by combing the hair with that fluid. The chlorine is readily detected by its odour, even after washing the hair as many as fifty times with water; while the tint is peculiar, by no means uniform, and not easily confounded with any natural colour; and the hair itself is hard, stiff, and brittle. Better results are obtained with nitric and nitro-muriatic acid, which, diluted with 50 times their bulk of water, impart a golden tinge to dark hair, without apparently injuring its texture. Peroxide of hydrogen has also been largely employed by hairdressers for this purpose. All these processes occupy time; and the fraud is easily detected by chemical tests; by allowing the hair to grow or even by stripping the person, and comparing the hair of the head with that of other parts; but the **fact must not be overlooked** that frequently considerable difference in colour naturally exists.

Change from light to dark.—The following methods have been adopted :—

a. Charcoal and grease.—This soils the fingers; and on placing a lock of the hair in hot water, the grease swims, and the charcoal falls to the bottom.

b. Salts of bismuth, lead, and silver.—The hair, freed from its oil by liquor ammoniæ, is moistened with a solution of one or other of these salts, and then, for a quarter of an hour, with sulphuretted hydrogen water. The black sulphides thus formed may be detected by steeping a lock of the hair in dilute nitric acid, and testing for the base. More than one of our photographic processes would effect the same change.

A mixture of litharge, chalk, and lime, in nearly equal proportions, dissolved in water (the *Tinctura Pompeiana* of the shops) was found very effectual. The hair was kept moist with it for three or four hours, and then allowed to dry. The chalk and oxide of lead were next removed with dilute acetic acid, and, lastly, the hair was rubbed with yolk of egg. The colour of the hair was thus effectually changed without injury to its texture. By steeping a lock of the hair in dilute nitric acid, the chalk is dissolved with effervescence, and with the lead converted into a soluble nitrate. Nitrates of calcium and lead remain in solution.

The hair undergoes marked change of colour in the course of some processes of manufacture. In turning rollers, for instance, out of the wood known as " green ebony," light hair assumes a green tint; a similar change results from working in an atmosphere containing finely-divided copper.

The effect of sudden and violent emotions of fright and grief in turning the hair grey has been much disputed, although numerous instances have been quoted, of these Mary Queen of Scots and Marie Antoinette may be mentioned; a like change may be produced by disease and other causes which are somewhat obscure. In a case related by Dr. Gordon Smith, a complete change of colour in the hair of the whole body took place in a single night in a girl 13 years of age, without previous indisposition or emotion; and Dr. Anstie (" Neuralgia and its Counterfeits," p. 94) has shown that, during attacks of facial neuralgia, the eyebrows and hair of the side affected sometimes turn grey, and even white, but resume their usual colour when the pain ceases. These changes in the colour of the hair are sometimes permanent, but the colour may in other cases be restored. When the hair of the head is the seat of the change, it is sometimes limited to certain portions only.

Identification by footprints.—It often happens that footprints are found on the soil, or the mark of a blood-stained foot on the floor of the spot where a bloody assault or a murder has been committed; and it may be of importance to compare the marks with the naked feet or shoes of the person suspected of the crime. As regards prints of the naked foot in the soil, a question naturally arises as to whether they can be taken as exact measurements of the foot itself, inasmuch as they must needs vary with the position and pressure of the foot and the character of the soil. But when the impression is that of a foot resting firmly on a tenacious soil, a comparison with the foot of the suspected person may be made with confidence; for it is highly improbable that the foot should yield the same mould in any two persons. When the feet of a suspected person present some notable peculiarity or deformity, the inference drawn from the comparison with the print gains greatly in force. Marks* of different size and shape are made by the same foot in running, walking, and standing. This shows the necessity of carefully comparing the impressions left on the soil with those made by the suspected person under similar conditions. In order to preserve footprints for future reference, it has been recommended by Hugoulin to heat the footprints with a hot iron, or chafing-dish, and dust powdered stearic acid over them. The hot iron or chafing-dish should be reapplied after each addition of the powdered stearic acid, and in this way the imprint is stiffened and preserved, and available for identification for an indefinite period.

Footprints in snow may be preserved by taking a plaster cast from an impression of them in gelatine.

The marks of naked feet on floors may require to be cut out for future reference.

The impressions left by shoes must be treated with like caution; but the original form of the shoe, aided in some instances by the position of patches or nails, may afford very important and even conclusive evidence, as in a case related by Sir Walter Scott, in which the murderer of a poor imbecile girl was discovered and identified by the marks of the shoes of the culprit left on the clay floor of the cottage during the death struggle.

Mind and memory.—In the Tichborne case, as in that of Martin Guerre (p. 47), questions relating to the mental faculties, and especially the memory, played an important part. In the first-named case considerations based on the facts brought out at the trial are at least as conclusive against the Claimant as the person, stature, and physical marks. The life the Claimant led in Australia was not such as to raise the question of the possible effect of hardship and exposure, whether on body or mind. There was no emaciation of body, but the very reverse, and no failure of mental power. He laid claim to an excellent memory, and the most plausible parts of his case depended on its exercise; and the

---

* Ogston, "Lect. on Med. Jurisp." 1878, p. 63, gives figures of the respective marks so produced.

fact of his using this, his good memory, whenever its employment promoted his views, proved his glaring mis-statements as to matters in which he had received no instructions from others to have been the simple result of ignorance. The same memory that claimed to recollect the name of a dog, or the number of a trooper's horse, could not have failed when tested with the Christian names of his mother, the handwriting of his father, his place of birth, his Paris residences, the companions of his childhood and youth, the college where he was educated, the studies he pursued, the examinations he passed, the relatives in whose houses he was always a welcome guest, the agent with whom he was in constant correspondence, the lawyer who made his will, the friends who helped him, the gallant soldier who gave him his commission, and his long, painful correspondence with the mother of the lady he would have made his wife. Nor did the defendant profess to have forgotten any circumstances connected with the lives of Roger Tichborne and his relatives. Roger's mother signs her Australian letter H. F. Tichborne. He does not say that he has forgotten her Christian names, which Roger knew well, but for *Henriette Félicité* he substitutes the homely English names, *Hannah Frances.* Roger took leave of his dying grandfather, Mr. Seymour, at Bath. The Claimant does not pretend to have forgotten the event, but shifts the scene to Knoyle. It was therefore of the very essence of the Claimant's case that he should display a tenacious and accurate memory. It was by the pretended exercise of it that he gained all his adherents. To admit the loss of it would have been fatal to his case.

Roger Tichborne's native language was French. He continued to speak it in France up to the age of 17, and frequently in England up to the age of 25. He acquired English later, and spoke it to the last with a French accent. The Claimant could not speak or read French; but he spoke Spanish as a man who had spent eighteen months in South America might be expected to do. Assuming, again, the identity of the Claimant with Roger Tichborne, had anything occurred to utterly destroy his knowledge of French? There is but one answer. It had not. The Claimant spoke Spanish years after he had acquired it. What reason, then, could there be for his having altogether forgotten French if he had ever known it? The Claimant was singularly tenacious of the habits he had formed. We may therefore assume that he would have retained some trace of the strong French accent with which Roger Tichborne always spoke English,

What degree and duration of light are needed for identification?—That a very short duration of a brilliant light suffices for this purpose is shown by the case of a lady, on her way from India who awoke on a dark night, and heard some one stirring in her cabin. A sudden flash of lightning enabled her to see distinctly a man rummaging one of her trunks, and so to discern his features as to identify him next morning. Some of the stolen things were found upon him, and he acknowledged the theft.*

In the following case, the question arose whether the light of a pistol-flash would suffice to discover the face of the person firing :—

The Sieur Labbe, on a dark night in May, 1808, was riding with the widow Beaujean, attended by a servant on foot. The servant was wounded in the hand by a gun fired through a hedge bordered by a ditch; and both he and his master swore that they recognised the assassin by the light of the discharge. An accused party, who was arrested, tried, and condemned to death, appealed to the Court of Cassation; and Gineau, Member of the Institute, and Professor of Experimental Physics in the Imperial College of France, was consulted as to the possibility of identification in the manner described. Accordingly, Gineau, his son, Professors Dupuis and Caussin, and others, stationed at different distances, to witness the effect, caused several primings to be fired in a dark room. The light, strong but fuliginous, was so transient that "it was scarcely possible to see distinctly the form of a head, and that of the face could not be recognised." The experiments were then repeated in the courtyard of the college, the gun being loaded with powder, but with the same results. The sentence was reversed.†

These experiments did not convince Foderé, who thought that if the night were dark and the persons within six, eight, or ten feet of each other, identification was possible : and the results are certainly at variance with the opinions of persons accustomed to the use of firearms, as well as with our own experiments. We repeatedly recognised the face of a friend by the discharge, in the dark, of a gun close at hand. It may also be reasonably con-

---

* Montgomery : "Cyclopædia of Pract. Med.," Art. Identity.
† Quoted by Beck from the "Causes Célèbres."

tended that, under the excitement of surprise or fear, a person might have a quicker and more distinct perception than an experimenter. The question, then, is one which, however well illustrated by these, as well as by carefully-planned experiments as to the duration and amount of light requisite for the perception of known and unknown objects of different size and colour, and at varying distances, admits of satisfactory solution only by collecting cases of this class.

The following case occurred in England in 1799:—One Haines was indicted for shooting at Edwards, Jones, and Dowson, Bow Street officers, on the highway. Edwards deposed that, in consequence of several robberies near Hounslow, he, with Jones and Dowson, set off in a post-chaise one dark night in November, and were attacked near Bedfont by two persons on horseback, one of whom stationed himself at the horses' heads and the other at the door of the chaise. By the flash of the pistols he could distinctly see that the man at the chaise door rode a dark-brown horse, between thirteen and fourteen hands high, of a very remarkable shape, having a square head, and very thick shoulders, and altogether such that he could pick it out of fifty horses; he had since recognised it. He also perceived by the same flash of light that the man had on a rough shag-brown greatcoat.*

A few similar cases have occurred in England; and there is a French case to the same effect in the Introduction to Foderé's "Treatise" (note, p. 28).

II. IDENTITY OF THE DEAD.

After death by accident or violence, and in cases of exhumation, the medical man may be called upon to assist in identifying the entire body; to reconstruct one that has been cut to pieces, and the parts scattered; or to examine a skeleton or parts of it, in order to determine the sex, age, and probable stature of the person to whom it belongs.

By careful examination he may ascertain the sex, form some judgment of the age, and even guess at the trade or occupation by the muscular development, the skin of the palms of the hands and the nails (indicating hard work, or the reverse), and the presence or absence of tattooing, so common in soldiers, sailors, and

---

* Montgomery : "Cyclop. of Pract. Med.," Art. Identity.

criminals, so rare in others. Stains on the hands or clothes may also help to determine the employment.*

The following are examples of successful identification :—

Dupuytren identified a murdered man chiefly by a malformation of the hip-joint ; and by a like deformity MM. Laurent, Noble, and Vitrey, a corpse buried in a cellar at Versailles three years. The body of Maria Martin was identified eleven months after her death by the absence of certain teeth from the upper and lower jaw, and by signs of inflammation, with extensive adhesions of the pleura, answering to an attack of inflammation of the chest, from which she was proved to have suffered shortly before her mysterious disappearance. A doubtful case, tried at Edinburgh, was decided by a dentist, who produced a cast of the gums. The scanty remains of the body of the Marchioness of Salisbury, discovered in the ruins of Hatfield House, were also identified by the jaw-bone having gold appendages for artificial teeth ; and the identification of the body of Dr. Parkman (see p. 52) was assisted by the very peculiar formation of the jaw, and the correspondence of part of it with a cast taken by a dentist.

The body of Harriet Lane, the victim of Wainwright, though much decomposed after twelve months' interment, was identified chiefly by the presence of an old scar on the right leg caused by a burn with a red-hot poker (see page 98, note).

In some remarkable instances an imperfect sort of identification has been effected after long interment. The real burial-place of some distinguished person has become a matter of dispute, and a coffin, such as was likely to have been used, has been discovered containing the remains of a body. In such cases, when the interment took place several centuries before in a leaden coffin or wrapper, the soft parts, though retaining their form at the moment of exposure, disappear at once as a fine dust. But when the interment is more recent, the body may be completely identified. The finding of the remains of Henry IV. in Canterbury Cathedral, after the lapse of nearly four centuries and a half,† is an example of the first class of cases ; the identification of the remains of Charles I., after 165, and of the patriot Hampden, after 185 years, of the second class.

Identification of Charles I.—The face of the king, though

---

* See this subject treated in detail in the Manual of Briand and Chaudé.
† See Felix Summerly's "Handbook for Canterbury."

disfigured, bore a striking resemblance to the portrait on coins, busts, and paintings, and the fourth cervical vertebra was found smoothly divided transversely. As this case is an excellent illustration of the condition, after 165 years, of a body suddenly deprived of life, embalmed and interred in lead, the following brief particulars are added :—On removing part of the lead coffin an inner coffin of wood, much decayed, was exposed, and within this the body, wrapped in cerecloth, into the folds of which an unctuous matter, mixed with resin, had been poured, so as to exclude the air.

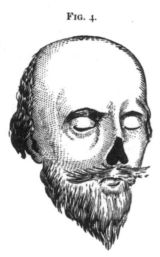

FIG. 4.

air. The coffin was quite full, and on removing the covering from the face, the skin was found dark and discoloured, the forehead and temples well preserved, the cartilage of the nose gone, the characteristic pointed beard perfect, the left ear entire, and the left eye open and full, though it vanished on exposure. The head was found loose, and was easily taken out and held to view. It was heavy and wet, with a liquid that gave to writing-paper and linen a greenish-red tinge. The textures of the neck were solid, and the back of the scalp was perfect and of a remarkably fresh appearance. The hair of the head was a beautiful dark brown, that of the beard of a redder tint. The divided muscles of the neck were considerably retracted, and the smooth surface of the divided vertebra was visible.

A reduced copy of the engraving which accompanies this description is annexed.*

In the same vault in which Charles I. was interred, Henry VIII. had been deposited. The leaden coffin, enclosed in a thick elm case, appeared to have been beaten in so as to leave an opening large enough to expose a mere skeleton of the king, with some beard upon the chin. The body had then been interred 266 years.

---

* "An account of the opening of the Tomb of Charles I.," in Sir Henry Halford's "Essays and Orations." The bodies of William Rufus, Henry I., Richard I., King John, and Edward I., have at different times been more or less completely identified.

IDENTIFICATION OF LIVINGSTONE.

The search for the body of Hampden was made on the 21st of July 1828, in the presence of Lord Nugent and others, in Hampden Church, Bucks. The coffin-plate being corroded, the coffin selected for examination was assumed to be his from its position near the tablet erected to his wife. It was of lead, and enclosed two wooden ones, of which the inner one was filled with sawdust. The body was tightly wrapped in three layers of cloth. The abdomen had fallen in. The face, white and marbled with blood-vessels, showed the upper part of the bridge of the nose, eyes but slightly sunk, auburn hair six inches long, strong whiskers, and some beard. The upper teeth were perfect, and those that remained in the lower jaw sound. The skull was well formed, and the forehead broad and high. The arms were muscular, the left perfect, but the right hand was detached, the bones of the arm having been sawn through. Several small bones of the hand, but no finger-nails, were found in a separate cloth. The nails of the left hand were entire. The socket of the left shoulder-joint was white; but the socket of the right shoulder was of a brownish tint, and the clavicle hung loose and detached from the scapula. The body measured 5 feet 9 inches, and was strongly built and muscular. The exhumation confirmed the account of Hampden's death as given by Sir Robert Pye, who married Hampden's eldest daughter, and at the same time went some way to explain Lord Clarendon's account of the shattered shoulder as the true cause of death. The dislocated shoulder was probably caused by a fall from his horse.[*]

A recent and most interesting case of identification is that of the great traveller, Livingstone. An ununited fracture of the humerus, the result of the bite of a lion, was sufficient identification in the case of the body of a European brought from the interior of Africa; coincidence being here quite out of the question. The remains were buried in Westminster Abbey.

Identification after very long periods of time is only rendered possible when the air has been excluded by close-fitting wrappers and sealed coffins. How the work of identification is interfered with by the march of putrefaction under ordinary circumstances of interment, and how it may be exceptionally assisted by conversion of the body into adipocere, will be shown when treating of putrefaction.

[*] " Annual Register " for 1828, Chronicle, p. 93.

To the preservation of the bones it is impossible to set any limit of time. Those of King Dagobert, disinterred from the Church of St. Denis after 1200 years, others from Pompeii after 1800, and others, as parts of Egyptian mummies, full 2000 years old, attest their permanence. There is, therefore, no medico-legal case in which they would not be found in a state fit for examination.

The cases of mistaken identity in the living have their parallels in the dead, as the following case will show :—

A resurrection-man was tried for raising the body of a young woman from the churchyard of Stirling, nine weeks after death. It was identified by all the relations, not only by the features, but by the left leg being shorter than the right. The jury was convinced that the *libel was proven*, and gave a verdict accordingly. " Now I am certain that this was not the body of the woman who was taken from the churchyard of Stirling, but one that, at least six weeks after the time libelled, was buried in the churchyard of Falkirk, from which she was taken by this man, who also took the other for which he was tried: she also was lame of the left leg. Thus, though guilty of the offence laid to his charge, he was found guilty by a mistake of the *corpus delicti*." (Dunlop, note to Beck's " Medical Jurisprudence.")

Cases illustrative of the possibility of dead persons being mistaken for living ones, not merely by acquaintances and friends, but by parents and near relations, are recorded by Smith, and by Dr. Cummin in his Lectures. (" Medical Gazette," vol. xix.)

Calculation of stature.—If we are dealing with an entire skeleton, we may calculate the stature of the person to whom it belonged by adding about an inch and a half for the soft parts. If the bones are detached, they should·be laid out as nearly as possible in the natural position, and then measured, making allowance, as above, for the soft parts.

It is commonly stated that, when the arms are stretched out horizontally, the line from one middle finger to the other is equal to the height. This, though inexact (and less true in women than in men), may be used to determine roughly the stature of a body of which only the bones of an arm are forthcoming. By doubling the length of the arm, adding twelve inches for the clavicles and an inch and a half for the sternum, as suggested by Dr. Taylor, a guess may be made at the stature.

M. Sue, more than a century ago, collected data for calculating the stature from the length of the extremities.* He measured a subject of medium height, chosen as well-proportioned. His measurements, reduced to English feet, inches, and lines, are given in the following table: the first three lines of which show the results of one measurement; the last two of averages:—

Age.	Body.	Trunk.	Upper Extremity.	Lower Extremity.
	Ft. in. lin.	Ft. in. lin.	Ft. in. lin.	Ft. in. lin.
1 Year . . .	2 0 0	1 2 5	0 9 7	0 9 7
3 Years . . .	2 11 3	1 8 4	1 3 0	1 3 0
10 Years . . .	3 1 0	2 1 7	1 8 4	1 9 11
14 Years . . .	4 10 8	2 5 11	2 4 1	2 4 10
20–25 Years . . .	5 8 2	2 10 1	2 8 0	2 10 1

According to M. Sue, towards the 20th, and from that to the 25th year, the upper border of the symphysis pubis forms the exact centre of the body, and so continues till in old age the spine becomes curved. Before 20, the centre of the body varies according to the age.

But Orfila, by measuring both the subject and the skeleton,† showed that Sue's statements must be received with caution. Thus, of 44 males (with 4 exceptions, adults), only 7 had the length from the vertex to the pubes exactly equal to that from the pubes to the sole of the foot; while in 23 instances the former measurement exceeded the latter; and in 14 fell short of it. The greatest difference on either side was $2\frac{1}{3}$ inches English. Again, in not one out of 7 females were the above measurements equal; the upper half of the body was longest in 6, shortest in 1. The males on an average were longer from the vertex to the pubes by more than $\frac{1}{3}$ inch, the females by $1\frac{1}{6}$ inch.

On examining the tables more closely, and bringing together the instances in which the length from the vertex to the pubes happens to be the same, we have found a considerable difference in the length from the pubes to the sole. Of 15 males measuring 2 feet 9 or 2 feet $9\frac{1}{2}$ inches from the vertex to the pubes, one measured as little as 2 feet 7 inches from the pubes to the sole, while another measured 2 feet $11\frac{1}{2}$—a difference of $4\frac{1}{2}$ inches. Again, of 5 females, in whom the upper measurement was 2 feet $6\frac{3}{4}$ inches to 2 feet 7 inches, one measured a little more than 2 feet

* "Sur les Proportions du Squelette de l'Homme." Mémoires présentés l'Académie Royale des Sciences, tom. ii. 1755.

† "Traité de Médicine Légale," tom. i. p. 105.

4 inches, the other less than 2 feet 8 inches—a difference of nearly 4 inches (G.).

So that in using Orfila's measurements, we might be in error to the extent of 4 to 4½ inches. His measurements of the skeleton exhibit deviations still more remarkable; for in one instance in which the upper part of the body measures 3 feet 1½ inches, the lower part measures only 2 feet 8 inches—a difference of 6½ inches; and in another, in which the upper measurement is 2 feet 5½ inches, the lower measurement is 2 feet 11½ inches—a difference in the opposite direction of 6 inches.

M. Sue's facts, then, are too few, and his statements too general, and even the more numerous and exact measurements of Orfila, if used to determine the stature, might lead to serious error.

Orfila's measurements of the cylindrical bones, which he used to calculate the stature of the skeleton and of the living body, also yield, as the subjoined tables show, very uncertain results:—

STATURE OF THE SKELETON, calculated from the length of the Cylindrical Bones.—(Orfila's second table.)				
LENGTH OF BONE.		STATURE.		
	Ft. in. lin.	Max. Ft. in. lin.	Min. Ft. in. lin.	Difference. In. lin.
Humerus (6 obs.) . .	1 1 0	6 1 3	5 9 9	3 6
Ulna 7 ,, . .	0 10 8	6 1 3	5 5 0	8 3
Femur 7 ,, . .	1 6 1	6 0 0	5 7 0	5 0
Tibia 7 ,, . .	1 3 0	5 10 6	5 5 0	5 6

So that for the same length of cylindrical bone we may have a variation in the stature of the skeleton of from 3½ to 8¼ inches.

STATURE OF THE BODY, calculated from the same data. (Orfila's first table.)				
LENGTH OF BONE.		STATURE.		
	Ft. in. lin	Max. Ft. in. lin.	Min. Ft. in. lin.	Difference. In. lin.
Humerus (19 obs.) . .	1 2 6	5 8 1	5 4 6	3 7
Ulna 14 ,, . .	0 10 8	5 10 10	5 5 8	5 2
Femur 12 ,, . .	1 5 9	5 9 8	5 4 6	5 2
Tibia 11 ,, . .	1 2 5	5 9 8	5 4 6	5 2

Here, then, for the same length of cylindrical bone, we have a variation in stature of from more than 3½ to more than 5 inches.

This minute analysis of Orfila's tables is rendered necessary by the undue importance he himself attached to them; for he says; "We are certain that it will be possible in the greater number of cases, on consulting these tables, and on having regard especially to the lengths of the femur and humerus, to arrive sufficiently near the truth." This false confidence arose from his not having made a proper use of his own figures; for it is obvious that, with such variations between the maxima and minima, calculations based only on averages cannot be applied to individuals with any degree of certainty. Dr. Henri Bayard, in three instances, in which the only parts of the body left were the bones, applied Orfila's data; in two unsuccessfully, but in the third with a success which is obviously due to a coincidence.

The following table shows the average measurements in English feet, inches and lines obtained from 44 male and 7 female subjects :—

	Stature.	Vertex to Pubes.	Pubes to Foot.	Upper Extremity from Acromion.	Femur.	Tibia.	Fibula.	Humerus.	Radius.	Ulna.
Male	5 6 6	2 9 6	2 9 0	2 5 6	1 5 8	1 2 7	1 2 2	1 0 5	0 9 5	0 10 2
Female	5 1 0	2 7 1	2 5 11	2 2 8	1 4 6	1 1 9	1 1 5	0 11 7	0 8 8	0 9 9

According to Humphry[*] the following stated percentages are the average proportions of the long bones in the adult European skeleton. Taking the full stature as 100, the spine measures 34·15; the humerus, 19·54; the radius, 14·15; the femur, 27·51; the tibia, 22·15. From these data, assuming them to be correct, the calculation of the stature from one of the long bones is a question of simple proportion.

AGE.

The law defines, with much minuteness, the privileges, immunities, and responsibilities that belong to the several periods of life. The medical man, however, is not often required to give evidence on this point; and the occasions for so doing will diminish as our registration of births becomes more complete.

[*] " The Human Skeleton," Table IV. p. 108.

It is chiefly as preliminary to complete personal identification that the question of age is important, and, like the general question, it divides itself into two parts—1. **THE AGE OF THE LIVING**; and 2. **THE AGE OF THE DEAD.**

I. AGE OF THE LIVING.

Human life has been arbitrarily divided into septennial and decennial periods, and certain ages (the climacterics) have been specified as epochs of unusual importance and danger. These divisions and distinctions are wanting in the precision necessary for medico-legal purposes.

Nor do the averages of Quetelet, based on the ascertained stature and weight of the body at different ages, admit of application to individuals, and the same objection applies to the position of the centre of the body as a test of age; for though it may be stated, in general terms, that at birth it is at the navel; in the adult, at the pubes; for intermediate ages, at intermediate points, nearer to the navel in the infant, and to the pubes in those approaching adult age; this statement is inexact, and especially in women, in whom, the thigh bones being shorter, and the trunk longer, than in men, the centre of the body is above the pubes.

The facts relating to the period of puberty in the two sexes, and of change of life in women, also show the little dependence to be placed on these occurrences as indications of age. The extremes are so far apart that the averages cannot be safely applied to individual cases.

We have more precise, though still very imperfect, means of fixing the age of younger persons, in the successive appearance of the teeth both of the first and second dentition.

The first set of milk-teeth, twenty in number, appear in the following order:—

Lower central incisors	7	months
Upper central incisors	8	,,
Upper lateral incisors	7–9	,,
Lower lateral incisors	10–12	,,
First temporary molars	14	,,
Canines	17	,,
Second temporary molars	22–24	,,

The milk-teeth, then, do not appear at the same age in all infants; while some are born with the incisors above the gums, others have no teeth till the end of the second year; and a few even live several years without a single visible tooth.

Nor do the teeth of the permanent set appear with such regularity in respect of time as to enable us to use the order and date of their appearance as certain tests of age.

The order and probable time of appearance of the permanent set, with the number of teeth existing at each age, is shown in the following table:—

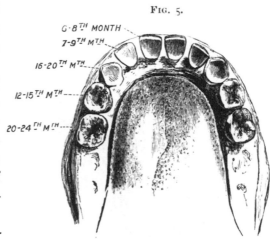

FIG. 5.

6·8TH MONTH
7-9TH MTH.
16-20TH MTH.
12-15TH MTH.
20-24TH MTH.

Temporary Teeth (Lower Jaw).

AGE.	INCISORS.		CUSPIDS.	BICUSPIDS.		MOLARS.			TOTAL.
Years.	Central.	Lateral		Anter.	Poster.	Anter.	Second.	Poster.	
7 ᴬᴹ	...	...	...	...	...	4	...	...	4
8 ᶜ ᴵ	4	...	...	...	...	4	...	...	8
9 ᴸ ᴵ	4	4	...	...	...	4	...	...	12
10 ᴬ ᴮ	4	4	...	4	...	4	...	...	16
11 ᴾ ᴮ	4	4	...	4	4	4	...	...	20
12 –12½ ᶜ	4	4	4	4	4	4	...	...	24
12½–14 ᵃ ᴹ	4	4	4	4	4	4	4	...	28
18 –25	4	4	4	4	4	4	4	4	32

As it was thought that the facts of this table might be employed as a standard of comparison in determining the age of children, especially of those employed in factories, Sir E. Saunders,[*] selecting the two periods of 9 and 13 years, observed the number of teeth existing at those periods in many hundred children, and obtained the following results:—

Of 457 boys 9 years of age, 219, or nearly one-half, had the number of teeth stated in the table; namely, 4 central incisors, 4 lateral incisors, and 4 anterior molars. Of 251 girls of the same

[*] "The Teeth a Test of Age." 1837.

age, 168, or much more than one-half, had the same number. Taking the two sexes together, 387 out of 708 had the full complement of teeth. The remainder in both sexes consisted of children who, in place of 4 of each kind, had a smaller number of one or the other. In a large proportion, one, two, or three of the four lateral incisors were wanting, and so of the other teeth; and in 52 cases the lateral incisors were absent.

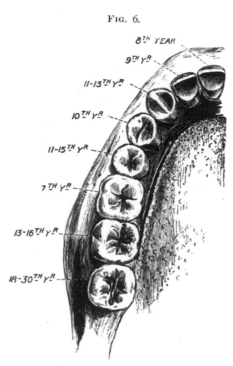

FIG. 6.

8TH YEAR
9TH YR
11-13TH YR
10TH YR
11-15TH YR
7TH YR
13-16TH YR
18-30TH YR

Permanent Teeth (Lower Jaw).

If, then, in the columns of the table, opposite the age of 9 years, we substitute for 4 the numbers 1, 2, 3, or 4, and assert that wherever any of these numbers are found, the child is in its 9th year, our assertion will be borne out in 656 out of 708 cases, or about 13 in 14. In the remaining 52 cases, a child of 8 might be mistaken for one of 9 years.

The inquiry respecting children who had attained the age of 13 gave the following results:—

Rather less than half the boys and more than half the girls, and as nearly as possible half of the two sexes taken together, had the full complement of teeth entered in the table as belonging to children of 12½ to 14; by far the majority of both sexes had one or more of the several orders of teeth; and in 11 instances only were some or other of the teeth wholly wanting. In three cases, a child of 13 might have been mistaken for one of 12 to 12½; in one case for a child of 11; and in one other for a child of 10. In a vast majority of instances, however, a child having one or more of the several teeth indicated in the columns of the table opposite 12½ to 14 years had completed its 13th year.*

* The results here stated in general terms were given in the first edition of this work in a tabular form.

The permanent teeth are not complete till the *dentes sapientiæ* make their appearance. This usually happens from the 18th to the 25th year, but sometimes much later; and a case is recorded by Dr. Hamilton of a man of 80 who died from the irritation produced by cutting a wisdom-tooth.

Some stress has been laid as a test of age on the white line at the margin of the cornea, known as the *arcus senilis*. As the arcus is occasioned by a deposit of oil-globules, which may take place from causes other than advancing age; as Mr. Canton reports cases of his own, or on the authority of others, in which it has been present at 42, 34, 33, and even at 28 years; and as we have ourselves seen it completely formed at 42 and 39, and absent at 79 and 85, it is obvious that this appearance must either be rejected as a test of age, or only used in healthy persons, living or dead, in conjunction with other signs of age (G.).*

All other indications of age in the living, such as grey hair or baldness, and loss of teeth, are deceptive. Cases of premature old age, of unusual vigour at advanced periods of life, and of restoration to the aged of some of the structures and functions proper to an earlier period (*e.g.*, the cutting of teeth and the growth of coloured hair; the secretion of milk, and the persistence or return of the menstrual discharge), may prevent us from even guessing at the age. On the other hand, the early occurrence of the marks of puberty in both sexes, and the premature or very late appearance of the menses in the female, create difficulties in rightly estimating the age at earlier periods.

II. AGE OF THE DEAD.

In the bodies of persons recently dead we have the same means of estimating the age as in the living, and we may learn something from the dissection of the body. Calcareous deposits in the heart and arteries, for instance, afford a strong probability that the subject had reached a mature if not an advanced period of life.

The state of ossification of the bones of the skeleton provides the best guide to the determination of the age. It would be out of place to enter into great detail here on this subject, for such information standard works on anatomy should be consulted, but

* "On the Arcus Senilis, or Fatty Degeneration of the Cornea." By Edwin Canton, F.R.C.S., *Lancet*, May 11 1851.

the following table, compiled mostly from Quain's Osteology may be found useful :—

A TABLE GIVING THE TIMES AT WHICH POINTS OF OSSIFICATION APPEAR AFTER BIRTH.

YEAR.	BONES.	YEAR.	BONES.
1st.	Lower segment of body of sternum.	**4th.**	Lower epiphysis of ulna.
	Small cornua of hyoid bone.		Scaphoid of tarsus.
	Coracoid process of scapula.		Great trochanter of femur.
	Head of humerus.		Upper epiphysis of fibula.
	Os magnum of carpus.		Middle cuneiform of tarsus.
	Head of femur.	**5th.**	Lesser tuberosity of humerus.
	External cuneiform of tarsus.		Internal condyle of humerus.
2nd.	Unciform of carpus.		Head of radius.
	Lower epiphysis of radius.		Trapezium and semilunar of carpus.
	Lower epiphysis of tibia.	**6th.**	Scaphoid of carpus.
	Lower epiphysis of fibula.	**7th.**	Trapezoid of carpus.
3rd.	Great tuberosity of humerus.	**19th.**	Olecranon process of ulna.
	Capitellum of humerus.	**12th.**	Pisiform of carpus.
	Pyramidal of carpus.	**13th–14th.**	Lesser trochanter of femur.
	Patella.	**14th–16th.**	Acromion process of scapula.
	Internal cuneiform of tarsus.	**16th–18th.**	Inferior angle of scapula.
		18th–20th.	Sternal end of clavicle.

The periods at which the ossification of the various parts of the skeleton is usually completed may also be of considerable practical value.

A TABLE GIVING THE TIMES AT WHICH THE DIFFERENT PARTS OF THE BONES UNITE.

YEAR.	BONES.	YEAR.	BONES.
1st.	Petro-mastoid and squamous portions of temporal.	**19th.**	Ilium, ischium, & pubes thro' acetabulum.
	Great wings & body of sphenoid.		Head & shaft of femur.
2nd.	Frontal bones.		Lr. epiphysis & shaft of tibia.
3rd.	Fontanelles completely close.	**20th.**	Upr. epiphysis & shaft of humerus.
4th.	Supra- and ex-occipitals.		Lr. epiphysis & shaft of radius.
6th.	Basi- and ex-occipitals.		Lr. epiphysis & shaft of ulna.
16th.	Coracoid process and body of scapula.	**21st.**	Lr. epiphysis & shaft of femur.
	Lr. epiphysis & shaft of humerus.		Lr. epiphysis & shaft of fibula.
17th.	Upr. epiphysis & shaft of radius.	**22nd.**	Occipital and sphenoid.
	Upr. epiphysis & shaft of ulna.		Upr. epiphysis & shaft of tibia.
	Smaller trochanter and shaft of femur.	**24th.**	Upr. epiphysis & shaft of fibula.
18th.	Internal condyle and shaft of humerus.	**25th.**	Acromion process & body of scapula.
	Great trochanter & shaft of femur.		Sternal epiphysis & shaft of clavicle.

Skull.—The separate bones of the skull are usually all united within a few years after birth. Occasionally, however, the two halves of the frontal bone remain separate through life.

Vertebral Column.—In the *third* year the arch and body of the vertebræ unite, and also the odontoid process and body of the axis. The epiphyses of the spinous and transverse processes commence to ossify about puberty, but are not united to the vertebræ till the age of *twenty-five* or later.

The individual vertebræ of the *sacrum* remain separate till the age of *eighteen*, when they begin to unite from below upwards, the process not being completed till the age of *twenty-five* or later. At a still later period, but subject to considerable variation, the coccyx becomes united to the sacrum.

Ribs.—The shaft and epiphyses of the ribs remain separate till the age of *twenty-five*.

Sternum.—The five segments of the sternum remain separate till the age of puberty, when the lower segments unite. The upper segments unite from the *twenty-fifth* to the *thirtieth* year. The manubrium and body do not unite till extreme old age.

Upper Limbs.—The various centres of the *scapula* unite from the *twenty-second* to the *twenty-fifth* year. The sternal epiphysis of the *clavicle* appears from the *eighteenth* to the *twentieth year* and becomes joined to the shaft at the age of *twenty-five*.

The head and tuberosity of the *humerus* unite at the age of *five*, and become joined to the shaft at the age of *twenty*. The condyles unite with the shaft from the *sixteenth* to the *eighteenth* year. The superior epiphyses of the *radius* unites with the shaft at from the *seventeenth* to the *eighteenth* year, and the lower epiphyses unites with the shaft at the age of *twenty*. The same holds in respect to the *ulna*.

The epiphyses of the *metacarpal* and *phalangeal* bones unite with their shafts about the *twentieth* year.

Lower Limbs.—The rami of the pubes and ischium unite about the *seventh* or *eighth* year; the various parts forming the acetabulum from the *sixteenth* to the *seventeenth* year, while the complete ossification of the os innominatum does not take place till the *twenty-fifth* year.

The head and shaft of the femur unite about the *eighteenth* or *nineteenth* year, while the lower epiphysis and shaft remain separate till the *twentieth* year.

The lower epiphyses and shaft of the *tibia* unite in the *eighteenth* or *nineteenth* year. The upper unites with the shaft in the *twenty-first* or *twenty-second* year.

The union of the epiphyses and shaft of the fibula occur somewhat later.

The epiphyses and shafts of the *metatarsal* bones unite from the *eighteenth* to the *twentieth* year; those of the *phalanges* about a year later.

If, then, on examination of a skeleton, or part of one, we were to find that bony union had not taken place at the points above indicated, we should conclude that the individual was under the age specified as that at which such union usually takes place; and at or over that age if ossification is completed. By careful examination of the state of ossification of the various regions, and comparison with more exact anatomical details, the age of the individual may be calculated with a considerable approach to accuracy within the period before the consolidation of the skeleton is complete. After that, that is, beyond 30, it is more difficult, and attention requires to be devoted more particularly to the signs of senile degeneration.

In old age there is a tendency to ossification of the cartilages of the ribs and larynx. Sometimes the larynx is entirely converted into bone. The bones become lighter, owing to absorption of the osseous plates of the cancelli. Hence the flat bones become thinner, through the approximation of the osseous laminæ. This is seen in the skull, scapula, and ilium. Owing to the same cause, the angle which the head of the femur forms with the shaft becomes reduced. The bones are more brittle, and more or less infiltrated with free fat, which gives them a yellowish colour and greasy aspect and touch. The sutures of the skull become less distinct or entirely obliterated. The intervertebral discs shrivel, the bodies of the vertebræ become bevelled off in front, and the spine bends forwards.

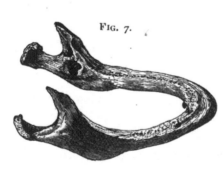

FIG. 7.

But the *jaw* is the part which changes most with age. In the fœtus and in early infancy the ramus and body form a very obtuse angle; in middle life, nearly a right angle; but in old age, when the teeth have dropped out, and the alveolar border is absorbed, it reverts to the infantile type. In very old persons the jaw has the characteristic appearance shown in the engraving (Fig. 7).

SEX.

This subject, like the foregoing, divides itself into two parts— 1. **THE SEX OF THE LIVING;** and 2. **THE SEX OF THE DEAD.**

I. SEX OF THE LIVING—DOUBTFUL SEX.

The question of sex may be raised in reference both to infants and adults. In the case of a new-born child, the issue of parents possessed of real or landed property, the right of succession, and, should it die, the disposal of the property, depends on the sex. If a wife, being tenant in tail male, is delivered of a son born alive, the husband's right is secured; but the property passes from him if she gives birth to a daughter. This form of succession is termed *tenancy by the curtesy.*

It may be necessary also not merely to ascertain the sex, where that can be done, but in doubtful cases, to determine which sex predominates; for it appears, on the authority of Coke upon Littleton, that "an hermaphrodite, which is also called Androgynous, shall be heire, either as male or female, according to that kind of the sexe which doth prevail, and accordingly it ought to be baptized."

The question of sex may also arise at a later period, as in the case, quoted by Beck, of a young nobleman of doubtful sex, whose parents consulted a medical man whether the education should be that of male or female.

There are three conditions of the organs of generation which may present difficulties to the medical examiner.

1. The organs of a male may resemble those of the female.

2. The organs of a female may resemble those of the male.
} False Hermaphrodism.

3. The organs of the two sexes may be blended.
} True Hermaphrodism.

1. The organs of the male may resemble those of the female (Androgyni). The most common malformation of this sort con-

sists of a small, imperfect, and imperforate penis, a short canal opening at its roof, and a cleft scrotum, bearing some resemblance to the clitoris, vagina, and labia of the female. Each section of the scrotum may contain a testicle, but the testes, one or both, may be lodged behind the external ring. The short canal, or *cul-de-sac*, which replaces the urethra and opens at the base of the penis, or in the perineum, near the anus, is found to communicate with the bladder. This opening is often enlarged, so as to resemble the vagina; and even to discharge its sexual function. From the position of the opening of the urethra beneath the imperforate penis these persons are called **hypospadians**.

The presence of testicles in the folds resembling the labia, or in the groin; the communication of the opening between the imperforate penis and the anus with the bladder; the absence of any organ corresponding to the uterus; and, in the adult, the absence of menstruation—enable us at once to determine the sex. In most of these cases the build of the body, the muscular development, the voice, the tastes and habits, are more those of a man than of a woman. Many cases answering to these descriptions are on record; and there are preparations, casts, models, and drawings illustrating these malformations in most of our museums. The following case by Mr. W. Loney (*Lancet*, May 7, 1856) is a good illustration:—Jane W——, a lunatic, 28 years of age, was admitted into the Macclesfield workhouse. She excited suspicion by her unwillingness to be washed, and on being examined was found to have a penis two inches long, and the same in circumference, placed on the pubes, just above and between the external labia; with a well-defined prepuce, which could be moved at pleasure, causing a slight erection. Just below this was an opening so small as scarcely to admit the little finger, and a ligamentous band could be felt at about three inches distance from its mouth. The urethra could not be seen, but a catheter was passed into the bladder through this opening. The penis was imperforate. The hair of the head was short and curly, like a man's; the limbs very muscular and hairy; and the voice exceedingly rough and masculine. The mammæ were entirely absent, and there was more hair than usual about the pubes. She had never menstruated. Her taste was so depraved that she would eat old poultices with great delight. She was strong and healthy, and annoyed the young women in the same ward by the display of her amatory propensities.

But there are cases in which an enlargement of the breasts, coupled with a preference for the society of the male, might mislead if the organs of generation were not examined; and in some instances the absence of the sexual passion creates uncertainty.

Sometimes the penis, well or ill formed, is confined to the scrotum by a peculiar formation of the integuments. This malformation, with the other deviations from the normal structure just described, occurred in two cases, one a Negro, the other a European, of which Cheselden gives engravings; and in the case of a child baptized and brought up as a girl, Mr. Brand, by a slight incision, liberated the restricted parts, and proved to the parents that they had been mistaken.

Another malformation belonging to this division, which might possibly give rise to doubt, consists in a deficiency of the anterior wall of the urinary bladder, and of the corresponding part of the abdominal wall, their place being occupied by an irregular, red sensitive mass, with the ureters opening upon it. The penis is short and imperforate, and the vesiculæ seminales open in a small tubercle at its root, or on the red and sensitive surface. The testicles are generally well formed, sometimes contained in the scrotum, sometimes to be felt in the groin, or they have not descended. The sexual appetite may be strong, weak, or altogether wanting. Those who have this malformation are called **epispadians.**

2. The female organs may resemble the male (Androgynæ). The malformations belonging to this class are an enlarged clitoris and a *prolapsus uteri.* In the first case—that of enlarged clitoris —the absence of testicles from the labia, the presence of a vagina and uterus, the occurrence of menstruation—these, singly or combined, render the distinction easy.

Cases of prolapsus uteri, involving a question of doubtful sex, have been recorded by Sir Everard Home and Mahon. Home's case was that of a Frenchwoman, who had *prolapsus* evident on inspection; she laid claim to the male sex, and was shown as a curiosity. Mahon's case is that of one Margaret Malaure, exhibited at Paris in 1693, dressed as a man, and alleging that she possessed and could use the organs of both sexes. Several physicians and surgeons certified that she was an hermaphrodite; but Saviard, an eminent surgeon, being incredulous, examined her in the presence of his brother practitioners, and found a *prolapsus uteri,* which he reduced.

3. The organs of the two sexes may be blended.

Many cases of this imperfect approach to true hermaphrodism are on record. In some an ovary has been found on one side and a testis on the other (lateral hermaphrodism); or the external organs have approximated closely to the female type, the internal to the male, or the reverse (transverse hermaphrodism).* But there is no case on record of the organs of both sexes perfectly developed in the same person; the nearest approach to this "lateral hermaphrodism" being the case of Catherine Hohmann, referred to in the note at the foot of this page.

In examining cases of doubtful sex, the following points should be attended to :—The size of the organ corresponding to the penis or clitoris, and whether it is perforate or imperforate ; the form and mode of attachment of the prepuce ; the presence or absence of parts corresponding to the nymphæ ; the presence or absence of testicles. If any opening exist it must be carefully examined with a sound, to ascertain whether it communicates with bladder or uterus, or is a *cul de sac;* and inquiry should be made respecting the existence of the menstrual or other vicarious discharge. The general conformation and appearance of the body should also be observed, including the growth of hair on the head, chin, and other parts ; † the formation of the shoulders and hips ; the development of the breasts ; the fulness of the thighs ; the tone of the voice ; and the feeling and conduct towards either sex.

II. SEX OF THE DEAD.

When the entire body is submitted to inspection, there should be no difficulty in determining the sex, except in those rare instances

* See the case of Durrje or Derrier in Cummin's " Lectures," *Med. Gaz.*, vol. xix. ; and for cases of the last-named malformation, occurring both in man and animals, the complete and learned paper on Hermaphrodism in the " Cyclopædia of Anatomy and Physiology." See also the case of Levi Suydam, respecting whom the question arose whether he was a male, and entitled to vote as a freeman, or a female (*Amer. Journ. Med. Soc.*, 1847) ; and the very remarkable case of Catherine Hohmann, who had the instinct both of the male and female, and who menstruated periodically, and had also seminal emissions containing spermatozoa (*Berlin. klin. Wochensch.*, Dec. 2, 1872 ; *Med. Times and Gazette*, June 28, 1873 ; and *American Journal of Obstetrics*, Feb. 1876, p. 615).

† The curious case given by Dr. Chowne of an otherwise well-developed female with copious beard and whiskers, cautions us not to attach too much importance to any single sign detailed in the text. For the case itself, and a learned history of similar instances, see *Lancet*, 1852, vol. i. p. 421.

in which the characters of the two sexes are blended; and in these, the sex, which could not be determined during life, may be ascertained by dissection.

But when the question of sex is raised after death, it is generally in reference to the skeleton, or some part of the osseous system, in which the following differences are observable :—

The bones of the female are lighter, more cellular, smoother, and less curved than those of the male; the processes less marked, and the joints smaller. The skull of the female is smaller, more ovoid, more bulging at the sides, and longer behind the foramen magnum; the face more oval, the frontal sinuses less strongly marked, the nostrils more delicate, the jaws and teeth smaller, and the chin less prominent. The chest of the female is deeper in its antero-posterior as compared with its transverse diameter than in the male; the sternum shorter and more convex; the

FIG. 8.

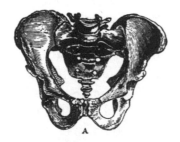 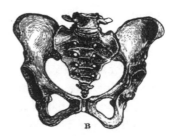

A   B

ensiform cartilage thinner, and ossified later in life; the ribs smaller, and the cartilages longer. The vertebral column is longer, and the bodies of the vertebræ are deeper in the female than in the male. The neck of the femur in the male forms an angle with the shaft of from 125° to 130°, whereas in the female the angle more nearly approaches a right angle. The pelvis, however, presents the most striking contrast. The ilia are more expanded and horizontal in the female; the sacrum more concave; the pubes more shallow; the angle formed by the descending rami more obtuse; the pubic arch wider, the tuberosities of the ischia more largely separated; the obturator foramen larger, more triangular, and more oblique; the acetabula wider apart; the entire pelvis more shallow, but larger in its outlets, than in the male. These differences are shown in the annexed engravings, in which A represents the male, and B the female pelvis.

The difference between the male and female skeleton is less strongly marked before the age of puberty.

The following table shows the respective measurements of the male and female pelvis at the brim :—

	Male.	Female.
Antero-posterior, or conjugate diameter	4 in.	$4\frac{1}{2}$ in.
Transverse	$4\frac{1}{2}$,,	$5\frac{1}{4}$,,
Oblique	$4\frac{1}{4}$,,	5 ,,

This group of subjects—Identity, Age, and Sex—may be advantageously brought to a close by three cases, one in the living and two in the dead, in one or other of which the question of identity in most of the forms it is likely to assume will receive ample illustration.

1. **The case of Martin Guerre.**—More than three centuries ago (in 1539) two children about 11 years old were married at Artigues, in Languedoc. The husband was Martin Guerre, the wife one Bertrande de Rois. After the lapse of nine years a son (Sanxi) was born under peculiar circumstances, known only to the parents. Martin, an elder son, lived with his father, but having robbed him, and fearing detection, disappeared, and was not heard of for eight years. In this interval the father died, leaving four daughters under the guardianship of a younger brother, Pierre. The absent Martin enlisted as a soldier, and had for comrade one Arnauld de Tilh (or Dutille) *alias* Pansette, a man of known bad character, who became so intimate with Martin as to possess himself of all his secrets. Martin lost a leg in the wars, and being taken ill, and thinking he should die, gave Arnauld what he had about his person. At the end of the eight years, this Arnauld, thus possessed of Martin's secrets and personal property, and having been mistaken for Martin by some friends of his, presented himself at Artigues, and was at once accepted as the real Martin Guerre by his uncle, sisters, and all his friends and acquaintance, and, most strange to say, by Bertrande herself, who, having been warmly attached to her husband, welcomed the new-comer with unfeigned affection, and bore him two children, one of whom died young. Arnauld lived with his comrade's wife, and surrounded by his comrade's relatives, friends, and acquaintance, for three years; when a soldier passing through the village startled Bertrande with the intelligence that her husband Martin, who had lost a leg in battle, was living in Flanders. Bertrande, disturbed but uncon-

vinced, went to a notary and bade him draw up a record of the soldier's statements; but she took no further notice of them, and continued to live with Arnauld as before. After three years, Pierre, the uncle, quarrelled with Arnauld, and would have killed him but for the interference of Bertrande. Soon after, in consequence of a village quarrel, Arnauld was arrested and imprisoned at Toulouse, and thereupon the uncle, with other relatives, tried to persuade Bertrande to denounce him as an impostor; but she resolutely refused, and when he was released on bail, received him as before with every mark of affection. But next day, the uncle, pretending to act under a power of attorney in Bertrande's name, arrested Arnauld on a charge of fraud and deception. When the case came on for trial, the uncle alleged that the prisoner was not Martin Guerre, but Arnauld de Tilh, known to many persons in the district from his youth as of bad character. On the part of the prisoner, on the other hand, all the facts connected with his early and complete recognition were adduced, and his perfect knowledge of matters the most trivial and the most secret, backed by Bertrande's upright character, blameless life, and strong affection. Witnesses, 150 in number, were then called, of whom between 30 and 40 had no doubt of the identity of the accused with Martin Guerre, 50 declared him to be Arnauld de Tilh, and 60, though on terms of close intimacy with both the parties, could come to no conclusion. The son, Sanxi, was then brought forward; and though no likeness could be traced between him and the prisoner, the latter was pronounced to have the family look, and bear the closest resemblance to the four sisters of Martin Guerre. The Judge, on summing up the evidence, gave sentence against the prisoner, as an impostor, adulterer, and usurper, and condemned him to be beheaded and quartered. But he appealed to the Parliament of Toulouse, which instituted a new inquiry. The prisoner, on being confronted with Bertrande, said he would abide by her decision, and place his life in her hands. Would she swear that he was not Martin Guerre? Bertrande answered "that she could neither swear nor believe it." Thirty new witnesses were then called, of whom ten swore that the prisoner was Martin Guerre, seven that he was Arnauld de Tilh; the rest spoke doubtfully. An uncle of Arnauld and some of his friends said they had recognised the prisoner as Arnauld from the first, but assigned reasons for not having exposed him.

The evidence of the witnesses as to the personal characteristics of the two men led to the conclusion that there was little resemblance between them. Martin was described as tall and dark, spare in body and limb, with his head sunk between the shoulders, a forked curved chin, a hanging lower lip, a large turned-up nose, an ulcer on the face, and a scar on the brow; while Arnauld was short, thick-set, and corpulent, had a stout leg and no stoop, a different set of features, and scars on the face about which the witnesses could not agree. But the prisoner had double eye-teeth in the upper jaw, a scar on the forehead, the nail of the fore-finger of the left hand sunk in the flesh, three warts on the right hand and one on the little finger, all which peculiarities were recalled by the witnesses as belonging to Martin Guerre. Martin's shoemaker deposed that his shoes had to be made a fourth longer than those of Arnauld. Martin, too, was a skilled fencer, which Arnauld was not, and Arnauld could not speak even a few words of Martin's native Basque language. One witness (Jean Espagnol, an inn-keeper) asserted that Arnauld had confided to him in the strictest secrecy all the facts relating to his close intimacy with Martin, and consequent knowledge of all his secrets.

The Parliament of Toulouse found the evidence conflicting. They attached great weight to the spontaneous recognition of Arnauld by those who might be presumed to be the best possible judges, as well as to his admitted resemblance to the four sisters of Martin; while, on the other hand, the lapse of time in the case of a lad who left his native village when only 20 years of age, added to the hardships and vicissitudes of a soldier's life, would serve, they thought, to explain even marked changes in form and face, and the failure to recollect the words of his native tongue, which, indeed, he might have forgotten before he left his native village. These considerations inclined them to give their sentence in the prisoner's favour. But at this juncture a man with a wooden leg, calling himself Martin Guerre, appeared in court. He was immediately arrested, shut up, and secretly examined, when he displayed the same knowledge of facts respecting his village acquaintances and family as Arnauld had done; and when confronted with the prisoner bore the test of cross-examination equally well, but often answering with less readiness, and even less minuteness of detail. The brother of Arnauld had absconded, and refused to appear. The new-comer was then brought face to face with members of the family of Martin Guerre. His sisters, as they entered one by one, glanced at him, threw their arms round his neck, burst into tears, called him their real brother, and asked his pardon a thousand times for having allowed themselves to be deceived; and Bertrande too, no sooner caught sight of him than she fell on her knees before him, urging in her exculpation of the wrong she had unwittingly done him, the astonishing resemblance between him and the villain who had deceived her, and the readiness with which his own sisters and all the villagers of Artigues had recognised him. The same revulsion of feeling showed itself in all who had borne witness in Arnauld's favour; and the judges, convinced by the tears and passionate grief of the loving wife, reinstated Martin Guerre in all his rights, and condemned Arnauld de Tilh to be hanged and burnt. Before his execution, the impostor made a full confession of his guilt.*

2, **Case of Houet.**—In the year 1821, Madame Houet, a widow lady, resident at Paris, disappeared; and Bastien, Robert, and Robert's wife, suspected of having made away with her, were tried before the Court of Assize, but for want of evidence set at liberty. In consequence, however, of information subsequently obtained touching a body said to have been buried about eleven years in a garden, the remains were so completely identified, and the manner of the death so clearly shown, that the prisoners were convicted and punished.

After excavating different parts of the garden, a workman hit upon a hollow spot, which was found to contain the remains of a human body, reduced almost to a skeleton. A drawing was made of the parts *in situ*. The figure lay on the left side, with the head bent on the neck, the vertebral column curved, and the right fore-

---

* We have retained this case, with a few slight abbreviations, as it stood in the fourth edition of this work; and we should have added the Tichborne case, but that we should have found it very difficult to bring it into a reasonable compass. It occupies thirteen pages in the Appendix to the fourth edition of this work, to which we refer our readers. The leading facts of that singular case will be found in sufficient detail in the text. We take the opportunity of here pointing out a simple procedure which, if put in practice, would guard against the occurrence of such scandals in future. The Home Secretary ought to be empowered in all such cases as the Tichborne claim, to appoint two or more skilled physicians and surgeons to make a preliminary report on the state of body and mind of the claimant; and unless a fair *primâ facie* case is thus made out, to refuse permission to engage in legal proceedings. Had the Home Secretary possessed and used this power, the Tichborne case could not have been brought into court.

arm raised, so that the hand nearly touched the face. The pelvis was turned obliquely upwards; the thigh-bones were raised, and the legs crossed beneath them. The prevailing colour of the remains was yellowish-brown, but the parts in contact with some of the long bones were of a deep-red tint.

The bones were small and delicate, those of the extremities not curved by muscular motion, and the marks of the insertion of the muscles few and faint. Among the bones of the left hand were found a small gold ring, carved in *facettes*; and several small well-formed finger-nails. The skull was small and oblong; the sutures well knit; the teeth white and well preserved; but three molars were wanting, and one of the incisors was carious. Some light-coloured hair was found, blended with grey hairs. The ossa innominata were largely spread out; the cavity of the pelvis not deep; the anterior part of the sacrum concave; the sub-pubic holes triangular; the cotyloid cavities wide asunder; and the upper opening of the pelvis had the diameter usual in well-shaped females. It was therefore justly inferred that this was the skeleton of a woman.

The third, fourth, fifth, and sixth cervical vertebræ, and right clavicle, were held together by a blackish mass, surrounded by several twists of a small decayed cord, leading to the inference that the deceased had been strangled, an inference fully borne out by the circumstantial evidence.

Several elaborate documents were drawn up by the reporters; of the first of which the following is a *résumé* :—

" 1. That these bones are those of a *human* skeleton. 2. That the skeleton is that of a *female*. 3. That she had attained the *age* of from 60 to 70. 4. That her height was about 4 feet 8 or 9 inches. 5. That her hair, which was a bright blonde in youth, was mixed with grey at the time of her death. 6. That the hands were small. 7. That during life the bones had suffered no injury. 8. That this woman died of strangulation, and that the act was, to all appearance, homicidal; and 9. That the body must have lain for several years in the earth."

The prisoners, who had long been suspected, were tried, condemned, and sentenced to forced labour for life.

3. **Case of Dr. Parkman.**—Dr. George Parkman, of Boston, U.S., was last seen alive on the afternoon of Friday, November 23, 1849, entering the Medical Institution in which Dr. John W.

Webster was Lecturer on Chemistry; and it was proved that he went there by appointment to receive money which Dr. Webster had long owed him. Dr. Parkman was missed, and could not be found; but on the Friday following his disappearance, in consequence of the suspicions aroused against Dr. Webster, search was made in his laboratory and the places attached to it, which issued in the discovery, in the vault of a privy, of a pelvis, righ thigh, and left leg, and some towels marked with Dr. Webster's initials, such as he was in the habit of using. There were also found in the furnace of the laboratory, mixed with cinders, many fragments of bone, blocks of mineral teeth, and a quantity of gold. A tea-chest was also found, which contained, embedded in tan, and covered with minerals, the entire trunk of a human body, the left thigh, a hunting-knife, and a piece of twine of the sort used in the laboratory. On the left side of the chest a penetrating wound was discovered; and to this the death was attributed. These portions of a human body being found in a medical college, it might be alleged that they were parts of a dissected subject; but this was shown not to be the case, for the vessels were free from all trace of the preservative fluid always employed in that college. They contained neither arsenious acid nor chloride of zinc. It

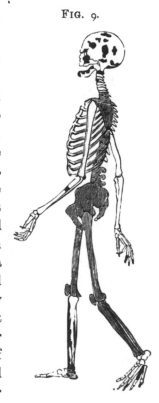

FIG. 9.

was further proved that the joints had been severed by a man having some anatomical knowledge and some practice in dissection. The fragments of the body, when put together, fitted accurately. The third and fourth lumbar vertebræ coincided; "the right thigh, on being placed in apposition with the pelvic portion, the bones, muscles, and skin, corresponded perfectly;" so also with the left thigh and pelvis, and the left leg and thigh. The fragments, therefore, belonged to the same body; and it was shown that there were no duplicate members or bones. By putting the parts together, and measuring them, they were found to be 57½ inches long; and adding three inches for the length from the outer malleolus to the sole of the foot, and ten inches from the crown of the head to the base of the sixth cervical vertebra, the length was brought up to 70½ inches, the exact stature of Dr. Parkman, as proved by his passport. As to his age, Dr. Stone stated that, judging from the skin, hair, and general appearance, the body belonged to a person from 50 to 60 years of age, and that the amount of ossification of the arteries would indicate that he was nearly or quite 60 years old. Dr. Parkman was about 60. The question of sex was not raised, as the parts of generation were found attached to the pelvis. Thirty-five fragments of bone were found, and among these three which, when put together, made up the greater part of the right hulf of the lower jaw, and enabled Dr. Wyman to ascertain that the teeth from the coronoid process to the first molar, or bicuspid, were wanting. To obviate this defect, a dentist had been applied to, not long before Dr. Parkman's death, to supply him with mineral teeth. These were found with the *débris* of the bones in the furnace, and the cast the dentist had taken fitted with great accuracy the very peculiarly shaped jaw of Dr. Parkman.

Thus the identification was complete; and, after a long and patient investigation, Dr. Webster was found guilty, and at length confessed the crime. He first struck Dr. Parkman on the head with a heavy stick, and then stabbed him in the chest.*

---

* This short account is taken from a full Report published at the time. Dr. Wyman exhibited at the trial a drawing of a skeleton with the bones that were found tinted yellow. In Fig. 9, taken from p. 54 of the Report, these fragments are printed black. The case affords a good example of the reconstruction of a mutilated body.

PART II.

CHAPTER I.

PERSONS FOUND DEAD—REAL AND APPARENT DEATH—SUDDEN DEATH—SURVIVORSHIP.

UNDER the general heading, persons found dead, the mode of conducting inquiries concerning persons whose manner of death is unknown, will be discussed. The first question in order is the reality of death; the subject of real and apparent death follows next; then sudden death, with the more common modes of dissolution; and lastly, survivorship.

PERSONS FOUND DEAD.

If sent for to a dying man, or to one already dead, the medical men must needs observe many things connected with the body itself, such as the position in which it is placed and the objects that surround it, which might be observed and stated in evidence by any common witness; but a post-mortem inspection, if required, must be entrusted to some skilled member of the profession. Hence the present inquiry has two divisions: 1. **THE RELATIONS OF THE BODY TO SURROUNDING OBJECTS.** 2. **DIRECTIONS FOR THE PERFORMANCE OF POST-MORTEM INSPECTIONS FOR LEGAL PURPOSES.**

I. RELATION OF THE BODY TO SURROUNDING OBJECTS.

As the medical man is summoned to most cases of severe illness or sudden death he is one of the first, as well as one of the best educated and most intelligent witnesses of those simple facts which in criminal cases constitute the presumptive or circumstantial evidence. He should therefore, especially in suspicious cases, attend to all that is passing around him, that nothing calculated to throw light on the cause of death may be overlooked. The following are the principal points to be attended to :—

Place in which the body is found.—This is not always that in which death took place, for both in suicidal and homicidal cases persons severely wounded may be able to move from the spot on which their injuries were received, and the murderer may try to conceal his crime by carrying the body to a distance. It must be remembered, however, that soldiers on the field of battle are sometimes found on the spot, and even in the very attitude in which they died.

Position and attitude of the body.—This may not correspond with the cause of death, as in the case where the body of a man killed by a blow on the head was found erect supported by a wooden fence; murderers also often so dispose of the bodies of their victims as to make it appear that they have committed suicide. The body of Sir Edmondbury Godfrey, who was proved to have been violently strangled, was found lying in a ditch, pierced with his own sword, and with his clothes so arranged as to create the belief that he died by his own hand; and persons have been poisoned, and afterwards suspended by the neck or thrown into water. If we find an expression of angry resistance on the face, hands, and body of the corpse, we may infer that death was the issue of a struggle; for while soldiers killed by gunshot often wear a singularly calm expression of countenance, those who have died in a hand-to-hand struggle often wear an expression of rage.

Spot on which the body is found.—In cases of fatal injury to the head it is usual to allege that the death was caused by a fall on some hard resisting body; an allegation only to be rebutted by an examination of the spot. A man found lying dead in a field with a severe bruise on the head, was alleged to have fallen on a stone or fragment of wood; but the field was carefully searched, and no such object could be found near the spot on which the body lay. In another case, a small wound of the head, which had penetrated to the brain, was attributed to a fall on a sharp object, such as a nail fixed in the floor; but the floor having been examined, and no such object found, it followed that the wound must have been inflicted by a small-pointed instrument. The murderer, who was acquitted through defective medical evidence, confessed that he had struck his victim with the point of a pair of snuffers.

Soil or surface on which the body lies.—Struggles often leave on the spot traces which may be compared with the clothes of the suspected murderer or of his victim, and footprints in the snow, or on the soil, have often furnished important evidence. In the case referred to at p. 25, the measure of the foot, the tread, and the mode in which the sole of one of the shoes had been patched, corresponded most closely with the foot-mark, and supplied the first link in the chain of evidence which led to the conviction of the murderer. In cases of murder, followed by the attempted suicide of the murderer, stains of blood have been found on the floor and on the soles of the feet of the perpetrator of the double crime.*

Position of surrounding objects.—In suicidal cases the instrument of death is generally found near the body; in homicidal cases it is often removed and concealed. In death by the more active poisons, the vessel which contained the poison is often found on or close to the person. The correspondence of wounds or bruises on a dead body with the objects immediately surrounding it, sometimes throws great light on the cause of death. The Prince de Condé was found suspended by the neck in his bedroom, and the correspondence of certain abrasions on the legs with a heavy chair placed close to them, and of others on the shoulder with a

---

* I was indebted to the late Dr. James Reid for the following instructive case given as nearly as possible in his own words :—"I was sent for one day to a man and his wife, whom I found lying in the same room with their throats cut. The woman was on the floor, with her right arm extended under the bed, and a razor close to her right hand. Her throat was deeply cut from ear to ear, and she lay in a complete pool of blood. The husband, who was in bed, had a wound in the throat, which had merely divided the trachea without wounding any important blood-vessel, and without causing any great loss of blood. When questioned, he gave the following account :—In the middle of the night he was roused from sleep by receiving a wound in the throat from the hand of his wife. The shock, the wound, and the loss of blood together, had prevented him from making any resistance or giving any alarm. My suspicions were aroused, partly by the man's manner, and partly by observing the water in a basin standing in the room slightly tinged with blood. In endeavouring to find some confirmation of my suspicions a thought struck me. I turned up the bed-clothes, and found the soles of the feet covered with dried blood. This fact, which I stated at the coroner's inquest, was deemed conclusive, but the man died almost at the moment that the verdict was passed " (G.).

projecting part of the window to which he was suspended, harmonised with the struggles of a man suspended during life, and justified the opinion of those who attributed the death to suicide.

The clothes.—Having noted the place and spot on which the body lies, its position, and the objects by which it is surrounded, a more close inspection should be made of the body itself. The clothes may be soiled with mud, corroded by an acid, stained by blood or some animal secretion, or they may be torn or cut. The place and character of the stains, and the direction of the rents or cuts, should be carefully noted; and cuts which traverse more garments than one should be compared with each other, and with wounds found on the body; for a murderer may try to conceal his crime by cutting the clothes after he has wounded the body, and the wounds and cuts may not coincide. Criminals are being constantly identified through the correspondence of things found in their possession, or in places to which they have access, with those used in the perpetration of the crimes themselves. The bearing and conduct of persons in attendance on the sick, dying, or dead, should not be overlooked, especially in cases of suspected poisoning.

To what has now been said respecting persons found dead it may be well to add that neither examples nor rules can do more than suggest the sort of inquiries that may be needed. There is always great scope for individual judgment, foresight and decision.

II. EXAMINATION OF THE BODY—POST-MORTEM INSPECTION.

The medical man having discharged the duty of a common witness by noting all those points of presumptive or circumstantial evidence which may throw light on the mode and cause of death proceeds to the examination of the body itself. When it is that of some person unknown, those characteristics which may lead to its identification should be noted down, in accordance with the instructions given at p. 28. Those appearances which serve to denote the time of death (see p. 284) should next be observed, and then any external injuries the body may have received.

WEIGHT OF VISCERA, ETC.*

	Weight. Male. Female.	Measurements, Contents, &c.
Brain . . .	49½ ozs. | 44 ozs.	
Spinal cord . .	1 oz. to 1¾ ozs.	15 to 16 inches long.
Thymus (at birth) .	½ oz.	
Thyroid body . .	1 oz. to 2 ozs. (largest in females).	
Lungs {right . . / left . .	24 ozs. | 17 ozs. } / 21 ozs. } 45 ozs. | 15 ozs. } 32 ozs.	
Heart . . .	9½ ozs. | 8¾ ozs.†	About the size of the closed fist (5 in. × 3½ in. × 2½in.). Circumference 9·2 at widest part.
Orifices of the heart—		
Mitral . .	...	4 in. in circumference.
Tricuspid . .	...	4½ ,, ,,
Aortic . .	...	3⅜ ,, ,,
Pulmonary .	...	3½ ,, ,,
Stomach . . .	4½ ozs. | Slightly under 4½ ozs.	Length 10 to 12 in. Diameter at widest part when moderately full 4 to 5 in.
Liver. . . .	50 to 60 ozs. | 45 to 55 ozs.	12 in. × 4 in. × 2 in.
Spleen . . .	5 ozs. to 7 ozs. (May vary even in health from 4 to 10 ozs.)	
Pancreas . . .	2¼ ozs. to 3½ ozs.	
Kidneys {right . / left . .	4⅓ ozs. | 3⅜ ozs. / 5½ ozs. | 5 ozs,	
Supra-renal capsules. (each) . .	1 to 2 drachms.	
Ureters . . .	...	Length 14 to 16 in.
Prostate gland .	6 drachms.	
Testicles (together) .	¾ oz. to 1 oz.	
Uterus(unimpregnated)	7 to 13 drs.	3 in. × 2 in. × 1 in.
Ovaries (together) .	120 to 200 grs.	
Bladder . . .	...	Size subject to great variation. Probably rather greater in females than males.

* The weights are to be regarded as averages only.

† The weight of the heart bears a direct proportion to the weight of the body generally, and especially to the development of the muscular system. Thus a perfectly normal heart may weigh considerably more or considerably less than the weight stated.

The condition of the face, whether pale or cyanosed, is important. If wounds, bruises, or excoriations exist, their nature must be specified, and their extent determined by exact measurement. The neck, back, and limbs should be examined in search of dislocations or fractures ; the chest compressed, to ascertain whether blood, or any fluid, mixed with air or gas, escapes from the mouth or nostrils ; the cavity of the mouth inspected, in search of foreign bodies or stains of corrosive poisons ; and the anus, for poisons introduced into the body by that opening. In new-born children the orbits, fontanelles and nuchæ should be searched for minute wounds inflicted by pointed instruments ; and in women, the point of junction of the breasts (especially on the left side) with the skin of the chest, and the organs of generation, in search of poisons, corrosive acids, or wounds.

Post-mortem inspection.—The great rule to be observed in conducting post-mortem inspections for medico-legal purposes is to examine every cavity and important organ. Even when the cause of death is quite obvious, it is well to observe this caution ; for if any part of the body have been left unexamined, the objection may be made that the cause of death might have been found there, or some disease which would give a mortal character to an injury not otherwise fatal. The order in which the cavities are examined must depend mainly on the supposed cause of death. As a rule, the seat of injury should be inspected first, before the contents of the blood-vessels have been disturbed by the examination of other parts. Specific directions for post-mortem examinations in cases of rape, delivery, poisoning, infanticide, &c., are given under those heads.

REAL AND APPARENT DEATH.

The risk of being buried alive, which was never very great in England, has now disappeared, and is not likely to recur unless in the improbable event of some fatal epidemic rendering speedy interment expedient. But the question of real or apparent death may assume practical importance long before the usual period of interment arrives ; for in cases of suspended animation the adoption, neglect, or speedy abandonment of measures for restoring life must depend on the previous answer to the question—Is life really extinct?

On the Continent, and especially in France, the practice of early interment, and the Roman Catholic rite of extreme unction, which raised a serious impediment to the use of means for restoring animation, has given importance to this subject. Hence such distinguished medical writers as Winslow, Bruhier, and Louis, have written treatises upon it, and it has received some attention at the hands of Mahon, Foderé, and Orfila.

There are three forms of suspended animation which may be mistaken for real death—(1) **Syncope,** (2) **Asphyxia,** and (3) **Trance.**

(1) **Syncope.**—In the majority of instances the apparent death, about which so much has been said and written, was merely a prolonged faint, as is proved by the success attending the accidental employment of cold water and fresh air, the most efficacious means of restoring those who have fainted.

The efficacy of cold water is attested by Hippocrates in a case of fever; and by John Howard, who bears his personal testimony to the restoration of supposed victims of gaol fever, brought out for burial, on being washed with cold water.

Diemerbröck and Zacchias attest the efficacy of pure cold air in cases of plague. Well-authenticated instances of such recovery after small-pox are on record, as in the case of an infant daughter of Henry Laurens, the first President of the American Congress, suffering from this disease, and laid out as dead; but the window of the apartment, that had been closed during the illness, being thrown open, the fresh air revived her. Such cases were not rare before the time of Sydenham, who abolished the stifling system of treating eruptive diseases, especially small-pox.

There is nothing improbable, therefore, in the cases of recovery from apparent death alleged to have occurred at the touch of the scalpel, or under the flame of the funereal pyre.

(2) **Asphyxia.**—This is a form of suspended animation liable to be mistaken for real death, and only to be distinguished from it by the result of the means employed for the recovery.

(3) **Trance.**—Cases of suspended animation not answering exactly to the description of syncope or asphyxia, occasionally occur in females. The motionless and insensible state of the frame, the cold surface, and the apparent suspension of respiration, and

circulation, combine to produce a semblance of death, and to create a temporary difficulty even for the medical man.

The subject of real and apparent death would be incomplete if some notice were not taken of those cases in which a state of apparent death has been brought about by an effort of the will. That such cases have occurred there is no doubt. A minutely described and well-authenticated instance of this kind—that of the Honourable Colonel Townshend—is related by Cheyne in his "English Malady":

"He told us he had sent for us to give him some account of an odd sensation he had for some time observed and felt in himself; which was, that, composing himself, he could die or expire when he pleased, and yet, by an effort or somehow, he could come to life again, which, it seems, he had sometimes tried before he had sent for us. We all three felt his pulse first; it was distinct, though small and thready, and his heart had its usual beating. He composed himself on his back, and lay in a still posture some time; while I held his right hand, Dr. Baynard laid his hand on his heart, and Mr. Skrine held a clean looking-glass in his mouth. I found his pulse sink gradually, till at last I could not feel any by the most exact and nice touch. Dr. Baynard could not feel the least motion of his heart, nor Mr. Skrine discern the least soil of breath on the bright mirror he held to his mouth. Then each of us by turns examined his arm, heart, and breath, but could not by the nicest scrutiny discover the least symptom of life in him. This continued about half an hour. As we were going away (thinking him dead), we observed some motion about the body, and upon examination found his pulse and the motion of his heart gradually returning; he began to breathe gently and speak softly." This experiment was made in the morning, and he died in the evening. On opening the body nothing was discovered but disease of the kidney, for which he had long been under medical treatment, all the other viscera being perfectly sound.

This case of Colonel Townshend is not only curious, but instructive, for it shows that there is at least one state of system so nearly resembling death as even to deceive medical men, distinguishable from real death only by the continuance of animal heat, the absence of rigidity, and the success of the means of restoration. This fact also admits of practical application; for it teaches us not hastily to abandon the attempt to resuscitate those who have seemed to perish by syncope or asphyxia, by hæmorrhage, shock, sun-stroke, drowning, and the several forms of suffocation.

SIGNS OF DEATH.

Of the signs of death insisted upon by authors, some are trivial and inconclusive, others are of considerable importance, both as signs and as the means of forming a judgment of the time that life has been extinct. To the first class belong the (1) **Cessation of the circulation**; (2) **Cessation of the respiration**; (3) **Extinction of muscular irritability**; (4) **Absence of sense and motion**; (5) **The facies hippocratica**; (6) **State of the eye**; and (7) **State of the skin.** To the latter class belong (1) **Extinction of animal heat**; (2) **Cadaveric rigidity**; (3) **Hypostasis**; and (4) **Putrefaction.**

INCONCLUSIVE SIGNS OF DEATH.

(1) **Cessation of the circulation.**—If no pulse can be felt at the wrist, and the beat of the heart can neither be felt nor heard with the stethoscope, we may assume that the circulation of the blood has ceased, though some feeble movements of the heart may have escaped observation. The absolute cessation of the heart's action may be taken as a sure sign of death; but the difficulty is to ascertain this beyond the reach of doubt. It is not enough to feel for the pulse at the wrist, for, as in Colonel Townshend's case, even experienced medical men might be unable to detect the pulsations, and conclude that the heart has ceased to beat. The stethoscope must be applied by an experienced person for several seconds, repeated at short intervals, before it can be said with certainty that the heart has ceased to beat. But if the heart does not beat for five minutes, we may conclude that death is certain. The apparent death of the Indian fakirs is much more remarkable than that of Colonel Townshend; but there is no reason to suppose that in them the heart ceases to beat, though the vital processes may be reduced to the lowest ebb. It should be noted, however, that in the state of hybernation into which some of the lower animals pass, the cardiac beats are reduced in frequency to a remarkable extent. Thus, in the marmot, which under ordinary conditions has 80 to 90

cardiac beats per minute, the rate is reduced during hybernation to 8 to 10 per minute. Assuming that a state analogous to hybernation may occur in human beings, it would be advisable, in cases otherwise doubtful, to prolong auscultation for twenty minutes to half an hour before pronouncing definitely on the question.

Seeing the difficulty attending the use of the stethoscope by uninstructed persons, Magnus has proposed an ingenious method of ascertaining whether the circulation has ceased or not. A ligature is to be applied to a finger, when, if there is life, a bloodless ring shows itself round the seat of the ligature, and a gradually increasing redness and lividity in the part beyond.

(2) **Cessation of the respiration.**—The circulation and respiration are so connected that what is true of the one is likely to be true of the other. The tests of respiration—the looking-glass and feather held to the mouth, and the cup of water placed on the chest or abdomen—are at least as delicate as those by which we seek to determine the continuance of the heart's action. It is scarcely possible that respiration, however feeble, should escape detection by such means; yet in the case of Colonel Townshend the glass remained for a long period unsoiled, and no sign of respiration could be detected. Hence it may be inferred that the suspension of the respiration is not a sure sign of death; but the joint cessation of the respiration and circulation, properly ascertained, would prove the fact of death.

(3) **Extinction of muscular irritability.**—This test was first proposed by Nysten; it is a certain sign of death. If a healthy muscle be laid bare and tested by puncture or by electricity, and there is no contraction, the body is dead. The different muscles of the body retain their contractility for varying periods after somatic death. Those of the limbs remain contractile on the average for about three hours after death, but the trunk and abdominal muscles retain their excitability longer. If, therefore, on examination it should be found that the muscles respond to electrical currents, the conclusion would be drawn, either that the body was still alive, or that death was quite recent, probably only a few hours. In no case have the muscles in any part of the body retained contractility for twenty-four hours. Hence discovery of electric contractility in a body supposed to have been dead more than twenty-four hours would at once indicate that life persisted.

These signs are confirmed by the following, which, though not of themselves conclusive, support each other:

(4) **Absence of sense and motion.**—This is common to suspended animation and real death, and therefore uncertain. The combination is not rare in hysterical females and in the mesmeric slumber; but in these cases the functions of circulation and respiration go on uninterruptedly, often combined with a vibrating movement of the eyelid.

(5) **The facies hippocratica.**—This peculiar expression of countenance is shown in the sunken eye, sharp nose, pointed chin, hollow temple, prominent cheek-bone, projecting ear and wrinkled brow; the dry livid skin and the white powdered hair of the nostrils and eyebrows. It is a trivial and unsafe sign of death, open to the serious objections—1. That it is nearly always absent in cases of sudden death and in the victims of acute disease; 2. That it is present in the dying as well as the dead, and even in cases that recover; 3. That it may be brought about by a strong impression of danger, the apprehension of a dreadful punishment, or the anticipation of certain death; and 4. That where it exists, it does not long survive the extinction of life.

(6) **State of the eye.**—A tenacious glairy mucus on the conjunctiva, causing a loss of transparency, and a collapsed and wrinkled cornea, are among the best and earliest of the trivial signs of death. But they are not conclusive; for, on the one hand, the conjunctiva may be invested by a mucous film and the eye grow dim in the living, and, on the other hand, in death from *apoplexy*, *carbonic acid*, and *prussic acid*, the eyes may continue brilliant and prominent for a long time. Putrefaction, too, or a ferment introduced into the stomach, by distending the body with gas, sends blood to the head, and makes the eyes brilliant and prominent. (Nysten.)* Owing to the cessation of the circulation, the eyeball loses its tension, and the fundus, if examined with the ophthalmoscope, is seen to have a yellowish-white hue instead of the rosy tint of life.

* Larcher [1] attaches some importance to a cadaveric imbibition of the sclerotic, which at a variable period after death begins to show a dark discoloration, first on the external aspect, and afterwards on the internal aspect of the globe, the two spots gradually growing so as to form the segment of an ellipse with the convexity downwards.

[1] *Archives Gén. de Med.*, June, 1862.

State of the skin—*Pallor*, owing to absence of circulation; *livid discolorations*, due to the subsidence of the blood; and *loss of elasticity*, have been mentioned among the signs of death. Pallor may exist during life, and be absent in several forms of death, especially in death from suffocation; and livid discolorations are common in aged and feeble persons in depending parts of the body. But loss of elasticity is a valuable sign, and one very early developed.

Among the trivial signs of death, the flexure of the thumb across the palm of the hand may be mentioned. It assumes this position before cadaveric rigidity comes on, but it is similarly contracted during life in certain spasmodic affections. The immobility of the pupil, the absence of vital reaction in the skin to irritants, &c., can only be regarded as of value when taken in conjunction with the more important indications above mentioned.

The foregoing signs do not supply the means of determining how long life has ceased. But the extinction of animal heat, rigidity, and putrefaction, being both certain signs of death, and means of determining, with more or less precision, the time at which death took place, must be examined more closely.

SIGNS OF DEATH WHICH ARE ALSO MEANS OF DETERMINING HOW LONG LIFE HAS BEEN EXTINCT.

(1) **Extinction of animal heat.**—The temperature of the body is closely dependent on the circulation of the blood; so that when this ceases, in a part or in the entire frame, that part, or the whole body, soon becomes cold. Hence the extremities grow cold before death, and even the internal parts, as is shown by the coldness of the breath; and at length, when life is extinct, every part becomes cold. But as, on the one hand, great coldness is often present during life and in cases of suspended animation, and, on the other, after sudden and violent death, the body often parts with its heat very slowly, the value of this sign is limited. Mere superficial coldness, as in collapse, must not be mistaken for death cooling, for there may be a high internal temperature with a very low external one. After death the body parts with its internal heat by radiation, so that the superficial temperature may rise above that which existed before death. Usually there is no further generation

of heat when life is extinct, but in certain cases, as in death from cholera, yellow fever, and some cerebro-spinal diseases, the temperature of the dead body has been observed to rise considerably above the normal temperature of life (as high as 113° F.), and Mr. Savory has shown that in a rabbit and dog killed by strychnine the temperature rose one or two degrees after life was extinct.

Nor is the extinction of animal heat a sure means of determining the time of death; for the rate of cooling varies with the age, the cause of death, the treatment of the body itself, and the state of the atmosphere; so that the period of cooling may vary from two or three hours to fifteen or twenty, and may even extend to upwards of four days.

The body cools slowly when clothed and exposed to a warm, still atmosphere; quickly when exposed, naked, to a draught of cold air. It parts with its heat more speedily in water than in air. Age, emaciation, and death by hæmorrhage or chronic disease, favour the cooling; youth and vigour, corpulence, and acute disease or speedy death, retard it. In persons dying of the same disease the extinction of animal heat is, *cæteris paribus*, as the rapidity with which it proves fatal. In chronic diseases the body parts with much of its heat during life.

Some important medico-legal cases which have occurred (cases of Hopley, 1860, Doidge, Gardner the sweep, and Jesse M'Pherson, 1862) have shown the necessity of examining this subject more closely, with a view, if possible, of determining the rate of cooling of the dead body and the time of death. Drs. Taylor and Wilks have recorded a series of observations on bodies transferred from the wards of Guy's Hospital to the dead-house. Out of 100 observations so made, 70 are available for a philosophical inquiry, and the facts, when submitted to careful examination and analysis, are found to yield some instructive results. The bodies, when removed from the wards to the dead-house, were placed in an open shell, and covered only with a shirt, shift, or sheet; and from the time of deposit in the dead-house the temperature of the skin of the abdomen was ascertained at various successive intervals by the thermometer. Seventy complete observations, recording the temperature of the wards and dead-house as well as of the body, and extending from February to June 1863 gave for the wards a range from 50° to 68° Fahr., and for the dead-house from 38° to 59°. Though several of the observations extended to from sixteen to twenty hours, the body in no case fell to the temperature of the air, the nearest approach to it being in the case of a girl æt. 19, who died of phthisis, and in whom sixteen hours after death, the temperature of the body had fallen to 52°, that of the dead-house being 48°. It is clear, then, that the cooling of the body, even when covered only by a single layer of cotton or linen, is a very slow process, and that in the case of a body clothed or in bed, and in a room of moderate temperature, it would be unreasonable to expect the cooling of the body till the lapse of upwards of twenty-four hours at the very least. It ought also to be understood that the temperature of the body, when first ascertained two hours after death, in eighteen instances presented a maximum of 88°, a minimum of 76°, and a mean of 83°; also, that on an average the rate of cooling is about 1° per hour. If, then, in any case we assume the temperature of the abdomen at death to have been 90°, and the temperature of the air 60°, it would not be reasonable to expect the temperature of the abdomen to have fallen to that of the air till the lapse of at least thirty hours.* This is confirmed, among others, by the observations of Letheby,† who found in the bodies of adult males, with a surrounding temperature of 55–57° Fahr., the axillary temperature 14° Fahr. and the rectal temperature 18° Fahr. *higher* than the air, so long as twenty to twenty-four hours after death.

The observations of Taylor and Wilks have the disadvantage of not having been commenced for some hours after death, and the method of taking the temperature is not such as is usually followed during life. On this point we have further important observations by Goodhart,‡ and by Wilkie Burman.§ According to Goodhart, we should be justified, as a general rule, in assuming that the temperature (taken in the axilla) was about the normal average. Burman, from his observations on patients just dead, and lying in bed, covered with the usual night-dress and the bedclothes partially turned down, arrived at the conclusion that the average rate of cooling was 1⅘° Fahr. per hour. Taking the difference between the axillary temperature observed in any case

---

* On the Cooling of the Human Body after Death, by Dr. Alfred S. Taylor and Dr. Wilks: *Guy's Hospital Reports*, Oct. 1863, p. 184.

† Quoted in Woodman and Tidy's "Forensic Medicine," p. 17 (note).

‡ *Guy's Hosp. Rep.*, 1870.   § *Edin. Med. Journ.*, 1880.

and the normal 98·4°, and dividing it by 1·6, would give the number of hours that had elapsed since death. Thus, if the observed temperature in the axilla was 80°, then 98·4 − 80 = 18·4° cooled, which, divided by 1·6, would give 11·5 as the number of hours that had elapsed since death.

It is, however, necessary to note that both the observations of Goodhart and Burman indicate that the rate of cooling is relatively much greater in the earlier than the later hours succeeding death, and more especially if the temperature at the time of death should be abnormally high. This is in accordance with what we should expect—the greater the difference between the body and the surrounding medium the more rapid the tendency to equalisation. In the first three hours after death, therefore, the loss of heat may be from 2 to 4 degrees; while in the later hours, when the difference between the body and the surrounding atmosphere is less marked, the loss may be little more than 1 degree per hour.

The observations of Niderkorn,* accord in the main with the above. He gives as the average axillary temperature, 96·9° Fahr., 2–4 hours; 90·2° Fahr., 4–6 hours; 81·7° Fahr., 6–8 hours; 77·9° Fahr., 8–12 hours, after death.

The use of the thermometer may be very properly insisted on in every case, as much more satisfactory than the sensations of the observer; and it is not to be doubted that very incorrect inferences may be drawn from the sensation of cold as imparted to the warm hand of an observer on touching the hands or feet, the nose or ears, of a corpse recently dead. A man must have little experience of living bodies who does not know what a sensation of icy coldness may be imparted to a warm hand by contact with the hands or feet of another.

(2) **Cadaveric rigidity—Rigor mortis.**—For some time after somatic death the muscles retain their irritability, and contract if stimulated. The duration of this irritability does not as a rule extend beyond two or three hours, and when it ceases cadaveric rigidity sets in. Before, however, rigidity becomes marked, the irritability of the muscle may be restored by the injection of defibrinated arterial blood or aërated venous blood through the vessels.

The irritability lasts longer in a low temperature than a higher one. Muscles become rigid at high temperatures—46° C. in the

* "De la Rigidité Cadavérique chez l'Homme," 1872.

case of frogs, and 50° C. in the case of mammals, The heat rigidity is essentially the same as death rigidity. Rigor mortis is due to the coagulation of the muscle plasma and the formation of myosin or muscle fibrin.

The muscle, formerly very elastic, becomes firm and non-elastic. If the rigidity be overcome by forcible extension of the limb, it does not return. Comparatively little shortening takes place in the rigid muscle, and cadaveric rigidity occurs in all positions of the trunk and limbs without materially changing those positions. It is entirely independent of the nervous system, for it comes on in muscles whose nerves have been severed, and in paralysed limbs if the contractility of the muscles has not been previously lost.

Rigor mortis occurs in the various muscles in a certain definite *order*. It shows itself first in the neck and lower jaw, then in the face, next in the chest and upper extremities, and lastly in the lower extremities.* It disappears in the same order in which it sets in, so that the lower extremities may be found rigid, while the trunk and upper limbs have become relaxed. Rigor mortis gives way to putrefactive changes.

The **time of its occurrence** and length of **duration** are exceedingly variable. It may even set in before the heart has ceased to beat. On the other hand, it may be delayed for twenty-four hours or more, and it may last for a few minutes or for several days. It occurs on the average within six, and lasts from sixteen to twenty-four, hours.

The experiments of Brown-Séquard † have thrown much light on the causes of variation. From these researches it appears that whatever exhausts or depresses the muscular irritability during life, favours the early occurrence of rigidity. Exhaustion of the muscles by repeated electrical shocks, or by violent muscular exertion, causes rigidity to appear early. It sets in rapidly in animals over-driven or hunted to death, in soldiers killed late in battle, and persons exhausted by convulsions (Savory). Though as a rule there is a period of relaxation before rigidity sets in, it would seem that under certain circumstances the muscles become rigid and fixed in the exact position assumed at the moment of death.

* The order stated agrees with the various observations of Casper, Nysten, Sommer, &c. ; but Larcher ("Acad. de Med.," June 1862) thinks the lower extremities become rigid before the upper.

† Relations between Muscular Irritability, Cadaveric Rigidity, and Putrefaction : *Proceedings of the Royal Society,* 1861.

The tetanic spasms of strychnine poisoning have been observed to pass directly into cadaveric rigidity.

This immediate setting in of rigor mortis has sometimes been termed "cadaveric spasm." It is not an unusual occurrence in cases of violent and sudden death, especially when there has been great nervous excitement. It has been specially observed in some cases of death in battle, in which the very attitude and expression at the moment of death are retained, and weapons are found grasped in the hand. And as the soldier will be found grasping his rifle in the act of taking aim, so will the suicide or murdered person be found clutching the object he held the moment before. This fact is of great importance from a medico-legal point of view. Thus, a razor or pistol found firmly grasped in the hand of a dead man is of itself a strong presumption of suicide, for it cannot be successfully imitated by a murderer.

Rigidity sets in early after death by lingering diseases, accompanied by general exhaustion, such as continued fevers, consumption, cholera, scurvy, and the asthenia of old age. In the feebly developed muscles of new-born children rigidity sets in early.

On the other hand, rigidity occurs late in cases of death in full muscular vigour. It is slow in showing itself in death from apoplexy, hæmorrhage, wounds of the heart, decapitation, injury of the medulla, and also in death by asphyxia. So also in death by rapidly fatal affections, such as acute inflammation of the viscera from irritant poisons, provided they have no specific action on muscular tissue.

As regards its duration, it may be stated as a general rule that if it sets in early it passes off quickly, and if it sets in late it lasts long. To this, however, there are some very important exceptions.

In some cases it which it sets in and passes off quickly it has been supposed that cadaveric rigidity does not occur at all. Hunter believed that in death from lightning rigidity does not occur. This, however, is by no means true, for in many cases of death from lightning rigidity is well marked, and bodies are not unfrequently found rigid in the attitude in which they were struck. In some cases, however, it may have set in and passed off so quickly as not to attract observation. It is said to be absent in some cases of narcotic poisoning (Casper), and in many cases of death from poisoning by mushrooms (Maschka). In many cases in which rigidity sets in early it entirely disappears in the course of one or two hours.

In those cases in which rigidity is delayed it often persists for several days. Thus in a case of suffocation observed by Nysten rigidity did not set in for sixteen hours, and lasted seven days. Similarly, Brown-Séquard found that rigidity in cases of death from asphyxia or decapitation did not set in on the average for ten or twelve hours, and lasted more than a week, even when the weather was warm. Taylor relates a case where the body of a man who died of apoplexy was exhumed three weeks after, in the month of January. Even at that period the limbs were so rigid that it required considerable force to bend them. A low temperature is favourable to the persistence of rigidity; so also, according to Casper, is recent indulgence in spirits. In those cases where rigidity lasts longest it may be found to co-exist with putrefactive changes.

As exceptions to the rule, that when it sets in early it passes off quickly, must be mentioned the rigidity of strychnine poisoning and many cases of cadaveric spasm. In these, though it sets in early, rigidity is often extremely pronounced and persistent.

Cadaveric rigidity can scarcely be confounded with the rigidity of freezing, or with tonic vital contraction. A frozen body is uniformly stiff throughout, and crackles if gently bent; whereas in cadaveric rigidity there is always a certain degree of mobility at the joints.

The rigidity present during life in such diseases as catalepsy and tetanus is readily distinguished from cadaveric rigidity by forcibly bending the limb—a limb rigid from vital contraction resuming its position when left undisturbed; whereas, cadaveric rigidity, once overcome, does not return. Rigor mortis occurs in the organic as well as in the voluntary muscles. The ventricles of the heart become rigid as a rule within an hour after death, and remain in this condition for ten or twelve hours, or longer; the rigidity giving place to flaccidity. These conditions have sometimes been mistaken for abnormal vital changes in the walls of the heart.

Rigidity, then, is a certain sign of death, and not to be confounded with any state of the living body; and as it supervenes after the extinction of muscular irritability, it is a sure indication of the hopelessness of attempts at resuscitation.

(3) **Cadaveric lividity, or hypostasis.**—This, too, is an infallible sign of death, scarcely requiring to be distinguished from any condition of the living body.

In the interval between the extinction of life and the commencement of putrefaction the body falls more and more under the influence of purely physical laws. The skin loses its elasticity and the flesh its firmness, and the blood, which was equally distributed, now gravitates towards the most depending parts. Hence the paleness of some parts and the deep violet tint of others, the discoloration of the occiput and back, and of the lowest lying parts of the intestines, lungs, and brain. These discoloured patches begin to form, on an average, from eight to twelve hours after death, and their seat is determined by the posture of the body. If it be placed on the face, they will occupy the anterior part of the body and of the viscera; and after hypostases have formed on the back, if the body be turned while still warm, and before the blood has coagulated, they will disappear. These discolorations are often very extensive, and when the body lies on a smooth surface, uniform in tint; but if the surface is uneven they are interrupted and irregular. The pressure of the clothes produces the same effect, so that a careless observer might mistake the marks of clothes fastened round the neck for the effect of strangulation, or isolated patches for severe bruises.

The extent and amount of discoloration are proportioned to the quantity of the blood, so that its prevalence through the whole body indicates a general fulness of the vascular system, and *vice versâ*. Sudden death, unattended by loss of blood, is characterised by extensive lividity, but lividity is not absent even in cases of death from hæmorrhage.

This subsidence of the blood explains the diminished intensity of colour in parts which had been the seat of the less severe and more diffuse forms of inflammation. But the appearances produced by such acute inflammation as follows burns and scalds, blisters and strong friction, and the action of the more violent irritant poisons on the internal parts, are permanent, and quite distinct in the dead body.

Cadaveric lividity must not be mistaken for ecchymosis or extravasation into the cutaneous tissues, the result of injury. They are easily distinguished from each other by making an incision into the discoloured spot. In hypostasis the cut surfaces will exhibit a few *puncta cruenta*, or bloody points, which are the open mouths of small blood-vessels; while in ecchymosis the blood will be found diffused into the cutaneous tissues. After some time, however, in hypostasis, the blood corpuscles become disintegrated, and the hæmoglobin transudes through the vessels, staining the surrounding tissues.

As hypostasis consists simply in the gravitation of the blood, whether in the skin or in the viscera, it is important, when it occurs in the internal parts, that it should not be mistaken for inflammation, as has happened in reference to the brain, lungs, and intestinal canal.

In connection with this subject of the subsidence of the blood, we must notice the coagulation and consequent separation of the constituents of the blood which takes place after death. This subject, recently much investigated by physiologists, was ably treated by Sir James Paget in a paper published many years since,[*] in which he shows that the blood contained in any cavity or vessel of the body at the time of death coagulates as it would do if drawn into a basin or other vessel during life; that the part of the blood which occupies the highest position in the body (like the buffy coat of blood in inflammation drawn during life) is least coloured, and that which lies lowest, most; that such highest portion may be like a nearly colourless jelly, while the lowest has a deep blue or black colour; that this post-mortem separation is distinguishable from similar separations during life, inasmuch as the latter adhere in layers (as in the sac of an aneurysm) to the containing cavity or vessel; and lastly, that in most cases the blood does not coagulate in the body till the lapse of from four to six, eight or more hours, but yet coagulates within a few minutes of being let out of the vessels. Sir James shows that these phenomena of post-mortem coagulation may have a practical application in determining the posture in which the body was left for some time after death; and he gives in illustration the case of a man suffering from excessive dyspnœa, who died in a sitting posture, with his head resting on his knees, and so remained for three or four hours after death. The relative position of the constituents of the coagula, the reverse of that usually observed, justified the

---

[*] On the Coagulation of the Blood after Death: *London Medical Gazette*, vol. xxvii. p. 613.

opinion expressed before the facts of the case were known to Sir James, that the body had not been laid out in the usual manner.

Besides these discolorations, due to the blood following the course of the vessels, there are others due to transudation. Thus the parts in contact with the gall-bladder are deeply tinged with bile.

(4) **Putrefaction.**—The chronological sequence of the phenomena characteristic of putrefaction, both (*a*) externally and (*b*) internally, has been minutely described by Casper, and may afford some indication of the time that has elapsed since death.

(*a*) **External phenomena.**—The first sign is the well-known greenish discoloration of the abdomen, which may take place in from **one to three days** after death, when also the eyeball becomes soft, and yields to the pressure of the finger. After **three to five days** the green coloration has become deeper, and spread over the entire abdomen; the genitals present a dirty brown-green appearance, and large or small patches of green make their appearance on other parts, particularly on the back, lower extremities, neck, and sides of the chest. Gas is developed in the abdomen, and forces a quantity of bloody froth from the mouth and nose. In about **eight to ten days** the discoloration has become darker, and the strong odour of putrefaction is well developed. The abdomen is distended with gas. The cornea has fallen in and become concave. The sphincter ani is relaxed. In certain parts of the body the cutaneous veins are seen as red cords in the midst of patches of paler colour. **Fourteen to twenty days** after death the body has become greenish-brown throughout; the epidermis is raised and peels off in patches; the abdomen and thorax are blown up; and the cellular tissue is inflated, so that the body has a gigantic appearance, and the features are completely obliterated. The penis is enormously swollen. The nails are loose and easily detached. The hair is also loose and easily pulled out.

The subsequent progress of putrefaction varies with the temperature and the medium in which the body lies. Thus a body far advanced in putrefaction, " at the expiration of one month, cannot with certainty be distinguished from one (*cæteris paribus*) at the end of three to five months." (Casper.)

The next stage is that of Colliquative Putrefaction.

The thorax and abdomen have burst. The sutures of the skull

yield. The orbits are empty, and the liquefied tissues leave the bones exposed. These separate, the ligaments being at length destroyed.

(*b*) **Internal phenomena.**—These first show themselves in the mucous membrane of the larynx and trachea, which, in from three to five days in summer, and six to eight days in winter, assumes first a dirty cherry-red or brownish-red colour, and then an olive-green.

The rate of putrefaction in the internal organs varies greatly.

TABLE SHOWING ORDER OF PUTREFACTION.

Putrefy Rapidly.	Putrefy Slowly.
1. Larynx and trachea.	10. Lungs.
2. Brain of infants.	11. Kidneys.
3. Stomach.	12. Bladder.
4. Intestines.	13. Œsophagus.
5. Spleen.	14. Pancreas.
6. Omentum and mesentery.	15. Diaphragm.
7. Liver.	16. Blood-vessels.
8. Adult brain.	17. Uterus.
9. Heart.	

Casper.

The stomach.—In from **four to six** days after death dirty-red patches appear on the posterior wall, and gradually extend over the whole interior. The mucous membrane becomes soft and pulpy. These changes are sometimes mistaken for the effects of corrosive poisons.

The intestines follow next, and then the **spleen**; then the **liver,** which, however, may retain its firmness for some months after death: putrefaction commences with a green colour on the diaphragmatic surface. The **brain** follows next. It collapses after death, and putrefaction commences in the line of the vessels. In two or three weeks it becomes quite diffluent. In children, however, the brain is the first organ destroyed by putrefaction. The **heart** and **lungs** putrefy more slowly, so that traces of disease are distinguishable in them long after they are quite decomposed. Orfila detected pneumonia 37 days and signs of pericarditis 57 days after death. The **kidneys** resist putrefaction longer even than the heart and lungs; the **bladder,** the **œsophagus,** and the **pancreas** resist still longer; and the **diaphragm** may be distinguished even after four to six months. The **uterus** resists putrefaction longest of all, and enables us to distinguish the sex after the complete destruction of all the other soft parts. Casper found it at the end of **nine months** in a fit state for examination, so that he could solve the question whether the deceased died pregnant, when all the other viscera were gone and the bones almost separated from each other.

Modifications of the putrefactive process.—I. **Adipocere or Saponification.**—Instead of passing through the various stages just described, the tissues may be converted into a soapy substance known as **adipocere**. This peculiar transformation was first observed by Fourcroy, at the end of the last century, during the removal of bodies from the Cimetière des Innocents at Paris. Adipocere has an appearance intermediate between fat and wax; hence its name. It is white or brownish, soft and unctuous, becoming whiter and harder when dried, and then remains for many years unchanged. It is an ammoniacal soap formed by the union of a fatty acid from decomposing fat with the ammonia given off by the decomposition of the nitrogenous tissues. Occasionally the ammoniacal base is replaced by calcium, so as to form a lime soap, especially when the body lies in a calcareous soil, or exposed to water containing calcium salts in excess.

In fully formed adipocere there is no change of structure, though fragments of unsaponified tissue may be mixed with it.

Adipocere is chiefly found in the fatter parts of the body, and in largest quantity in the corpulent, since the fat rapidly decomposes, yielding fatty acid; but it is probable that muscle and other tissues are transformed into adipocere, so that the fatty acid is also developed from the decomposition of the albuminoid constituents of the body. Hoffman considers, however, that it is probably formed only from fat; the muscles disappearing by colliquative decomposition. The bodies of children undergo the transformation more quickly than those of adults.

It is rare for the whole body to become saponified; but many bodies were found completely transformed, and of a dead white, among the large number of bodies disinterred while laying the foundations of King's College Hospital; and pure white specimens of the brain, and of the contents of the orbits, will be found in the museum of King's College. Saponification also takes place, more or less completely, in the bodies of fœtuses that have undergone maceration in the womb (see p. 116), and Casper relates a case where the whole of a fœtus became thus saponified *in utero*.*

Water is necessary for saponification, so that the process only takes place in bodies which have lain in water or in a damp soil. As to the length of time required no fixed rules can be laid down. It was formerly wrongly supposed that a period of thirty years was necessary for the transformation of a body; but Devergie states that one year is required if the body is in water, and about three years if buried in a damp soil. Casper thinks that adipocere is not likely to form to any considerable extent in less than three to four months in water, or half a year in moist earth, though it may be commenced at a much earlier period. In some cases it may be observed in the space of five weeks in bodies floating in water, (Taylor.)

2. **Mummification.**—Another condition presents itself under certain peculiar circumstances. Instead of undergoing colliquative putrefaction or saponification, the body becomes dried up or *mummified*—a name which sufficiently indicates the appearance the body assumes. It is desiccated throughout, the soft parts being retained, but converted into a hard, dry, husky-looking substance, closely adhering to the bones. The odour is that of old cheese rather than that of putrefaction. The change occurs when the body is subject to conditions which rapidly abstract moisture from the tissues, as in the dry sands of the desert, or when exposed to heat and currents of dry air. It is also said to occur in arsenical poisoning, the poison acting as an antiseptic, and opposing the putrefaction changes.

Some of the bodies disinterred in laying the foundations of King's College Hospital presented only bones covered with skin, to which in parts the hair adhered. A specimen of this sort was varnished, and placed in the museum of the College.

If we would infer the time of death from the progress which the putrefactive process has made, we must pay special attention to the causes which affect it.

Causes affecting Putrefaction: (1) External, (2) Internal.

1. **External.**—These are: (*a*) **Temperature**, (*b*) **Moisture**, (*c*) **Access of Air**, (*d*) **Time of Interment**.

(*a*) **Temperature.**—Putrefaction is arrested by a temperature of

* Casper, " Ger. Med.," 5th ed. vol. ii. p. 42.

212° and of 32° F.: the higher temperature dries it by evaporation; the lower congeals its fluids and delays the development of bacteria. The most favourable temperature is one ranging from 70° to 100°; one, indeed, most favourable to the growth of organisms. Putrefaction therefore takes place more rapidly in summer than in winter, and, other things being equal, varies with the temperature.

(b) **Moisture.**—This is an essential condition, without which putrefaction cannot begin, or, having begun, continue. The body contains in all its parts moisture enough to ensure decomposition; but such parts as the brain and eye, which contain most fluid, are most prone to putrefaction; dropsical subjects also putrefy speedily. Putrefaction also commences soon, and runs a rapid course, in inflamed parts, in bruises, and at the edges of the wounds.

Bodies which have remained some time in the water, and are then exposed to the air, putrefy more rapidly than those that have not been immersed; but in bodies which remain in the water putrefaction goes on slowly.

On the other hand, a dry air retards or arrests putrefaction. Hence the preservation of the bodies of travellers on sandy deserts. A rapid current of air has the same effect by promoting evaporation; but a moist and stagnant atmosphere encourages it, both by retarding evaporation and supplying moisture.

(c) **Access of air.**—That the presence of air promotes putrefaction is shown by the slow development of gas that takes place when blood or flesh is introduced into a vessel through mercury, so as to exclude all the air which does not attach to the substance introduced; also, on the other hand, by the preservation of flesh in gases not containing oxygen, such as hydrogen and nitrogen; and less completely in those in which oxygen is chemically combined with some other gas, as in carbonic acid and nitrous acid; again, in atmospheres filled with vapours that absorb oxygen, such as turpentine. Oxygen, taken separately, promotes putrefaction more than any other gas, but when mixed with nitrogen, as in the atmosphere, its activity is greatly increased. The free access of air also affords the most favourable condition for the access of the minute organisms which are the active agents in the putrefactive process.

Heat, moisture, and free access of air, then, are the conditions most favourable to putrefaction ; and in judging of the time at which death took place, we must weigh well the amount of influence each of these agents has brought to bear on the result.

(*d*) **Time of interment.**—Bodies putrefy much more speedily in air than in the ground. Hence the longer interment is delayed, the greater the changes they undergo. Thus, during summer a body exposed for five or six days, and then interred, undergoes at the end of a month as much change as it would do at the end of seven months had it been interred at once. (Orfila.)*

(*e*) **Site and mode of interment.**—In dry, elevated situations putrefaction goes on slowly ; in low swampy grounds, rapidly. A dry absorbent soil retards putrefaction, a moist one accelerates it. In sand or gravel the change goes on slowly, and adipocere is rarely met with ; in marl or clay, and in loose mould, especially that which is impregnated with animal or vegetable matter, it proceeds more quickly (except peat, which retards putrefaction). The deeper the grave, *cæteris paribus*, and the more completely the body is defended from the air by clothes or coffin, the slower the putrefaction. It is rapid when the body is in contact with the soil, but very slow when buried in a coffin hermetically sealed.†

2. **Internal.**—(*a*) **Age,** (*b*) **Sex,** (*c*) **Condition of Body, and Cause of Death.**

(*a*) **Age.**—Other things being equal, the bodies of children putrefy more speedily than those of adults and aged persons, and the bodies of old persons more rapidly than those of adults.

(*b*) **Sex.**—According to Orfila, putrefaction is more rapid in women than in men. He attributes this to the greater quantity of fat they contain, an explanation which, though not quite satisfactory, agrees with the fact that the corpulent putrefy more readily than the lean and emaciated. Casper, who disputes the influence of sex, observes that the bodies of women dying during or soon after child-birth putrefy very rapidly.

(*c*) **Condition of body and cause of death.**—Putrefaction takes place most speedily in bodies filled with fluid. Hence it is very

---

* Reinhard, as the result of the examination of exhumed bodies in Saxony, states that in gravel or sandy soil the destruction of the soft parts in children is complete in four years ; in adults it is complete in seven years. In clayey soil the period is rather longer. See *Brit. Med. Journ.*, Feb. 10, 1883, p. 267.

† Consult Orfila's "Traité des Exhumations Juridiques," and Devergie's "Médicine Légale," which contains the marrow of Orfila's observations, with his own account of the changes produced by putrefaction in the water. See also Casper's Handbook.

rapid after sudden death and death from acute disease (*e.g.*, fifteen hours in a woman dying from hydrophobia in mid-winter— Sauvage); also after some cases of hyperpyrexia due to severe injury of the nervous system, as from fracture of the cervical vertebræ; slower after death from hæmorrhage or chronic diseases, unless complicated with dropsy, or extensive structural change, as in typhus and typhoid fevers, small-pox, erysipelas, septicæmia, &c.

What is true of the whole body is true also of its parts; for those which are full of fluid at the time of death, through inflammation, congestion, or dropsy, wounds or bruises, putrefy more rapidly than healthy and entire structures. In some instances, as in low fevers, the extremities are attacked before the trunk has ceased to live.

It was formerly believed that the bodies of persons killed by poison putrefied very rapidly; but this is now known to be a mistake. Casper specifies phosphorus, alcohol, and sulphuric acid, to which we may safely add arsenic and other mineral poisons, as retarding putrefaction, and though he classes smoke and carbonic acid with sulphuretted hydrogen and narcotic poisons, as hastening it, it appears from three cases reported by Devergie that in death by carbonic acid the process is decidedly retarded. Animal and vegetable poisons have probably no effect either way; persons killed by them putrefy rapidly, as in other cases of speedy death. Putrefaction takes place with unusual rapidity in animals driven soon after a meal and dying suddenly,[*] in men dying suddenly during violent exertion, and in soldiers killed late in battle.

Putrefaction in water.—More dependence is to be placed on the criteria laid down for determining the period of death of bodies which have remained in the water, than of those exposed to the air or interred, for the temperature of the water is more uniform, and the body, unless when it rises to the surface, is protected from the air. As Devergie, whose official position at the Paris Morgue gave him unusual means of observation, places much reliance on the signs by which the period of death is determined in the drowned, the following account, based upon his description, is subjoined:—

[*] See two striking illustrations of this—one in a pig, the other in a man—in my edition of Walker's "Original," p. 24 (G.).

The bodies of the drowned are subject, like those who perish in other ways, to loss of heat and rigidity, and to putrefaction, but in a modified form, being accompanied by the formation of adipocere. One of the first changes, which occurs as early as the **third or fourth day**, consists in bleaching of the skin of the hands. **At the end of a week** the body is found supple, and the skin of the palms of the hands very white. **A week to twelve days** of immersion bleaches the backs of the hands, and softens and bleaches the face. At the end of **a fortnight** the hands and feet are bleached and wrinkled, the face slightly swollen with spots of red, and the middle of the sternum has a greenish tint. At the end of **a month** the hands and feet are completely bleached and wrinkled as if by a poultice, the eyelids and lips are green, the rest of the face reddish-brown, and the front of the chest presents a large green patch with a reddish-brown spot in the centre. At the end of **two months** the face is swollen and brown, and the hairs are but slightly adherent: much of the skin of the hands and feet is detached, but not the nails. At **two months and a half** the skin and nails of the hands are detached, and the skin of the feet, but the toe-nails still adhere. In the female, reddish discoloration of the subcutaneous cellular tissue of the neck, of that surrounding the trachea, and of the organs contained in the chest. Partial saponification of the cheeks and chin; superficial saponification of the mammæ, the axillæ, and the fore part of the thighs. At **three months and a half** the skin and nails of the hands and feet are completely removed; part of the hairy scalp, of the eyelids, and of the nose, and the skin of many parts of the body destroyed; and the face and upper part of the neck and axillæ partially saponified. At **four months and a half** nearly total saponification of the fat of the face, of the neck, of the axillæ, and of the anterior part of the thighs, with commencing earthy incrustation; incipient saponification of the anterior part of the brain; opaline state of the greater part of the skin; almost entire separation and destruction of the hairy scalp; calvarium denuded and beginning to be very friable. For more remote periods no accurate approximations can be given.

Devergie alleges that the above signs have been repeatedly applied with complete success to the investigation of bodies that had been in the water for unknown periods.

The foregoing description applies to bodies immersed during winter. Bodies immersed in summer undergo the same changes much more rapidly. Thus, 5 to 8 hours in summer correspond to 3 to 5 days in winter; 24 hours to 4 to 8 days; 48 hours to 8 to 12 days; 4 days to 15 days. On the average, then, the same changes in summer take place from three to five or six times as rapidly as in winter, or even more promptly than that, the changes in spring and autumn being intermediate.

That development of gas within the body which causes it to rise to the surface takes place slowly in winter, and the body rarely floats in less than six weeks or two months. The same change takes place in summer from the 14th to the 16th day, or even earlier.

Of putrefaction generally, as a means of fixing the period of death, it should be observed that it is surrounded with difficulties, in consequence of the many elements that must combine to produce these changes in the body. So that we read without surprise the following statements :—" On the 20th March 1848 I examined the bodies of 14 men, almost all of the *same age*, 24–30 years, previously occupying precisely the *same social position* (workmen of the lowest class), all lying together in the *same* part of our deadhouse, who had all met the *same* death, having been shot on the barricades on the 18th of March, and had all notoriously died at the *same* time." " And yet I can testify that in no one case did the signs of putrefaction resemble those of another." " An old couple of about the same age (50–60 years) were suffocated during the night by carbonic acid gas. Up to the time of our examination these bodies had been exposed to precisely similar influences, and yet on the fourth day after death (in November) the body of the man was quite green, both on the abdomen and the back, and the trachea was brownish-red, from putridity, &c. ; while his uncommonly fat wife was perfectly fresh both outside and in." (Casper's Handbook, vol. i. pp. 33 and 34.) In the face of facts like these, we find both French and German authors speaking with much confidence of the value of the signs of putrefaction ; and even Casper himself stating that at a similar average temperature putrefaction in the open air, in water, and in a coffin, will have advanced equally after the lapse of one, two, and eight months respectively.

Sometimes this change produced by putrefaction involves questions of life and death, as the following case (Reg. *v.* Pile, Maidstone

Summer Assizes, 1891) will show. On or about the 22nd of March, 1891, an unmarried woman was delivered of a male child, the live birth of which was disputed. On that day she took the body from the house and on the 29th May following, the remains were found in a stable, below some manure. The weather between these dates had been generally dry and cool; when found, the head was extensively injured, the abdomen was green and the skin was peeling, the scrotum and penis (excepting the urethra) had disappeared, and there were remains of the testicles. It was first thought the child had only been dead a week, but Stevenson bore testimony to death being possible seven weeks previously. The woman was convicted of concealment of birth.

THE MODES OF DEATH.

The proximate causes of death, whether from natural decay, disease, or violence, may be reduced to two—viz,, cessation of the circulation and cessation of the respiration. On the continuance of these functions, and particularly of the former (if these may be specified where all are essential), the life of the body as a whole and of the individual organs and tissues depends. These functions may cease from causes operating directly on their mechanism, but also by causes operating indirectly through the nerve centres by which they are regulated. Hence it is usual, in accordance with Bichat's classification, to speak of three modes of death—viz., death beginning at the *heart*, death beginning at the *lungs*, and death beginning at the *head*. This classification is convenient, for though death beginning at the head is in reality death by failure of the circulation or respiration, or both, through affection of the vital nerve centres, yet the affection of the nervous system is the primary fact and the phenomena are sufficiently characteristic to deserve separate consideration. It must, however. always be borne in mind, that, owing to the interdependence of all the vital functions, there is no such sharp line of demarcation between the different modes of death as we make between them for purposes of classification.

1. **Death from failure of the circulation.**—This may be sudden, as in **syncope** and **shock,** or it may be gradual, as in **asthenia.**

(*a*) **Sudden failure of the circulation.**—For an efficient circulation it is necessary that there should be a sufficient quantity of blood, and a differential tension in the arteries as compared with the veins. The circulation will be brought to a standstill by any cause which greatly lowers the vascular tension or annihilates the differential pressure in the arterial system. The cause may be in the heart, or in the vessels, or both.

In the **heart.**—As the pumping action of the heart is the chief factor in the maintenance of the arterial tension, all organic or structural diseases which render it incapable of propelling its contents into the arterial system will naturally result in the cessation of the circulation, and death. Under this head are classed all diseases of the heart and its annexes, and especially aortic incompetency and fatty degeneration of the heart.

But apart from structural disease or degeneration, the heart may suddenly cease by nervous shock conveyed through the vagus nerves. The heart may be inhibited temporarily, or finally and for ever, by central nervous influence, as by emotion or blows on the head ; or reflexly, as by a violent blow on the epigastrium ; or by sudden irritation of the sensory nerves of the stomach, as in corrosive poisoning ; or even by swallowing a large quantity of cold water when the system is overheated.

Death from sudden cessation of the heart's action is death from **syncope.** Syncope, however, may be merely transitory, as in ordinary fainting. In syncope there is sudden loss of consciousness, owing to diminished blood-pressure in the cerebral centres. A deadly pallor overspreads the skin, with superficial coldness, and life may become extinct without any further symptom.

In the **vessels.**—Rapid fall of blood-pressure and cessation of the circulation will naturally result from great loss of blood owing to rupture of the vessels from injury, or disease such as aneurysm. This is death from hæmorrhage. But without actual loss of blood a vascular area may, under certain conditions, become so dilated, and the differential pressure so lessened, that the circulation ceases. This is what occurs in death from **shock** or collapse. From blows on the abdomen, or violent irritation of sensory nerves, the vascular area of the viscera becomes so dilated as practically to retain almost the entire volume of blood in the body. Hence, even though the heart may continue to act, yet little or no blood flows through it. The animal, as it were, dies of hæmorrhage into its own veins. This has been experimentally shown to occur in frogs from blows on the intestines. It is seen in cases of traumatic shock, more especially from abdominal injuries. The individual suffering from shock merely, still retains consciousness, and thus differs from one affected by syncope. Frequently, however, more especially from blows on the abdomen, there is not merely reflex dilatation of the abdominal vessels, but also temporary inhibition of the heart, so that syncope and shock coexist, and the individual is unconscious. But syncope may pass off, leaving the symptoms of shock remaining. Shock, like syncope, may be transient or fatal. In this condition there is pallor of the face and lips, superficial coldness, cold sweats, muscular relaxation and dilated pupil. The patient complains of giddiness, tendency to syncope if raised from the recumbent position, dimness of vision, ringing in the ears. The pulse is almost imperceptible, the respiration sighing and gasping. There is frequently nausea and vomiting, restlessness and tossing of the limbs, transient delirium and convulsions.

In death from failure of the circulation the post-mortem appearances vary according to whether the cause has been in the heart or vessels. Structural disease or fatty degeneration of the heart will reveal itself on examination. The cavities of the heart may be found full, the heart having been unable to contract on its contents. Inhibition of the heart without structural disease will not reveal itself by any special morbid appearances in the heart itself, though it is most likely to occur in a heart already weakened by degenerative processes. In reflex inhibition the heart stops in the state of diastole, but this may not be observable on post-mortem examination, as the heart may empty itself on the setting in of cadaveric rigidity.

In death from shock the heart is quite empty, and the blood accumulates in the abdominal veins. Death from hæmorrhage reveals itself in an unnatural pallor of all the internal organs, and an almost empty state of all the venous trunks. If the hæmorrhage has been internal, the blood will be found internally, and the ruptured vessels will in most cases be discoverable.

(b) Gradual failure of the circulation.—This may be termed death by asthenia proper, though the term is sometimes employed differently. It is the natural termination of life from decay, and is comparatively rare, death in the aged being frequently due to some intercurrent affection. It is also the mode of death after wasting and exhausting diseases, cold and starvation. The vital powers fail gradually, and life often passes away so quietly that it is difficult to say when the last spark has been extinguished.

2. **Death from failure of the respiration.**—This is termed death from **asphyxia**, which literally means pulselessness, but is generally understood to mean the condition that supervenes on interruption of the function of respiration. Attempts have been made to substitute for this the term apnœa, as being more exact, but this tends only to create confusion, as apnœa is employed by physiologists to signify a condition of cessation of the respiratory movements when the blood is artificially kept hyper-oxygenated, so that the respiratory centre is no longer stimulated by the blood. The older term asphyxia, though etymologically inexact, is yet sufficiently well understood.

Asphyxia may result from many **causes of obstruction to respiration.** They may be divided into two categories—**internal** and **external**.

Internal.—Under this head we may include paralysis of the respiratory nerve-centres from disease or injury of the medulla oblongata; injury or paralysis of the nerves or muscles of respiration—as by curara, coniïne, &c.; rigid fixation of the muscles of respiration, as in the tetanic convulsions of strychnine poisoning; collapse or disease of the lungs, rendering the lungs incapable of expanding or aërating the blood; occlusion of the pulmonary artery; air in the veins; occlusion of the air-passages by organic disease or spasm of the glottis, pressure of tumours, and the like.

External.—To this group belong occlusion of the air-passages by foreign bodies; pressure on the chest not capable of being overcome by the muscles of respiration, as in dense crowds, and even (as in a remarkable case on record) in taking a plaster cast of the chest; closure or pressure on the air-passages, as in suffocation, strangulation, hanging. These are all cases of obstruction of the respiration in a medium supposed capable of supporting life. To these are to be added conditions in which, though the respiratory movements are free, the surrounding medium is incapable of oxygenating the blood—viz., submersion in a liquid medium (drowning); or an atmosphere devoid of oxygen, such as hydrogen or nitrogen. These gases have a purely negative effect, but many other gases which are classed as asphyxiants, such as carbonic oxide, sulphuretted hydrogen, chlorine, &c., have positive toxic effects, besides being unable to support respiration. We may term such vapours *toxic asphyxiants*.

Phenomena.—When a warm-blooded animal is placed in an atmosphere devoid of oxygen, or in one not containing a sufficient proportion of this gas (under 10 per cent.), or when the mechanism of respiration is in any way obstructed, it begins to exhibit signs of agitation, and to make powerful expiratory and inspiratory efforts, during which all the accessory muscles of respiration are brought into action. The vascular tension increases, the superficial veins become distended, the surface livid, and the eyeballs protrude. The individual at this stage experiences a sense of fulness of the head, ringing in the ears, and various sensory illusions, sometimes of a pleasant character.

Soon total unconsciousness comes on, and the dyspnœic efforts pass into general convulsions, in which the muscles of expiration come more particularly into action, and in which the sphincters are forced and the excretions voided. On these convulsive efforts there follows a calm, in which the animal lies insensible, with dilated and immovable pupils, and reflex excitability abolished generally. All muscular movements cease, except those of inspiration, which are prolonged and are repeated at intervals. As death approaches these become shallower and irregular, and are succeeded by stretching convulsions, during which the back is straightened, the head thrown back, the mouth gapes, and the nostrils dilate. The heart continues to beat after all other movements have ceased, and ultimately stops in diastole. Death is then absolute.

Course and termination.—The time necessary to bring about a fatal termination varies. Excluding special considerations, it may be stated as the result of the Med.-Chir. Committee's experiments,* that when the respiration of a warm-blooded animal is totally obstructed, all external movements cease in from three to five minutes, and the heart stops within ten minutes. Certain modifications occur according to the method in which asphyxia is produced. (See Drowning.) It has been observed that the young of some animals resist asphyxia longer than the adults. The differences, according to Bert, depend on the relative activity of the internal respiratory processes. The

* *Med .Chir. Trans.*, vol. xlv. 1862.

greater the gaseous interchange the more rapidly fatal is obstruction of the respiratory functions.

Post-mortem appearances.—After death by asphyxia livid patches are seen on various parts of the body, and cutaneous hypostasis generally is well marked. The blood is dark and completely reduced. It remains long fluid, and coagulates very imperfectly. The venous side of the heart, the great venous trunks and pulmonary arteries, are gorged with dark blood, while the left side of the heart is completely empty, or contains only a comparatively small amount of dark blood. The lungs are sometimes congested, but this is by no means constant. Often, and especially if the respiration has been completely obstructed from the beginning, the lungs are pale at first, but become hypostatically congested after some time. The lining membrane of the air-passages is frequently injected, and coated with a sanguinolent froth. Punctiform ecchymoses may be seen on the surface of the lung, and some of the air-cells are distended or ruptured. The abdominal viscera are usually congested. The state of the brain varies. Sometimes it is found congested with numerous *puncta cruenta* and serous effusion, but there may be no abnormal appearance.

Various other signs characterise the special modes in which asphyxia has been brought about.

Pathology.—Inasmuch as asphyxia implies both a deficiency of oxygen and an accumulation of carbonic acid, the question has been debated as to which is the essential factor. The experiments of Pflüger, Rosenthal, &c., seem to demonstrate that the phenomena are mainly due to the oxygen starvation. But that the accumulation of carbonic acid has no effect at all cannot be maintained, for it is demonstrable that carbonic acid has a direct effect on nerve centres and living tissues generally.

The circulation of non-oxygenated blood through the lungs and respiratory centres in the medulla is the cause of the active respiratory efforts in the first stage, both by direct irritation and reflex stimulation. The respiratory movements increase in force, and the irritation of the respiratory centres radiates into the centres for other movements, giving rise to the expiratory convulsions ascribed by some to irritation of a so-called "convulsion-centre." These centres become ultimately paralysed, but the medullary centres retain their vitality after the brain and spinal cord have lost their excitability. Increased resistance is offered to the heart owing to the constriction of the systemic and pulmonary arterioles by the circulation of non-oxygenated blood and by the convulsive movements. The ventricles in consequence become distended, and the heart's action laboured. The heart also becomes enfeebled by the circulation of non-oxygenated blood in its walls, the diastolic intervals become longer, and it finally stops in the state of diastole with both cavities full of dark blood. On the setting in of cadaveric rigidity, however, the left ventricle usually succeeds in emptying itself, so that as a rule the right side is seen full, and the left empty and contracted.

3. **Death from paralysis of the vital nerve centres.**— Under this head we include those forms of death in which the functions of the brain are primarily interfered with, giving rise to **coma** and leading to death secondarily, by paralysis of the centres of respiration and circulation.

The causes of coma are numerous. It may be brought about by pressure on the brain, by fractures of the skull, effusions, hæmorrhagic or otherwise, or tumours. Or it may be due to the circulation in the blood of poisons—classed generally as the *narcotic* poisons—introduced from without, or of poisons generated in the system, as in uræmia and diabetes, and in other cases of non-elimination of waste products. Coma may come on gradually or suddenly, according to the cause. Affections of the brain causing coma—such as cerebral hæmorrhage, are rarely suddenly fatal. Sudden death occurs only when the effusion is at the base. In coma the individual lies in a state of unconsciousness, from which he cannot be roused. There is complete insensibility to external impressions, the breathing becomes stertorous and finally ceases, death occurring quietly or in convulsions.

The **post-mortem appearances in death from coma** are essentially those of asphyxia, which is the proximate cause of death ; but apart from structural changes (the cause of the coma), congestion of the brain and its membranes is more marked and constant than in death in asphyxia from other causes.

VIOLENT AND SUDDEN DEATH.

Upwards of 3000 sudden deaths occur year by year in England and Wales from causes not ascertained, over and above the 19,226 returned as due to violent causes, of which the greater number also belongs to this class.

The following facts relating to sudden death are taken from the 55th Annual Report of the Registrar-General. Of 559,684 deaths from all causes occurring in England in 1892, 19,226, or about 1 in 30, were violent deaths, of which 2892 were due to various forms of chemical injury, 5610 to asphyxia, 8967 to various mechanical injuries, and the remaining 1757 to other causes not stated. Of the 19,226 violent deaths, 13,570 occurred in males, and 5656 in females.

The suicides in the year 1892 amounted to 2583, of which 1907 were men, and 676 women. Of 2478 due to ascertained causes, 1255 were by various forms of suffocation, 301 by poison, 8 by burning, and the remainder by mechanical injuries; among which were 501 cut-throats, 261 gun-shot wounds, and 77 falls. The suicides by poison of men and women respectively were as 6 to 4, by asphyxia as about 3 to 1, and by mechanical injuries as about 5 to 1. The greatest number of suicides among the men occurred between the ages of 45 and 55, those among the women between the ages of 35 and 45.

According to Ogston,[*] the most common causes of sudden death, excluding violence and poison, are as follows :—1. Diseases of the heart, especially fatty degeneration, angina pectoris, aortic re-gurgitation, interstitial abscess, rupture of the heart or of its valves, and diseases of the pericardium. 2. Diseases of the blood-vessels, especially aneurism and thrombosis ; the aneurisms most likely to end thus suddenly are intra-cranial, intra-pericardial, abdominal, and pulmonary. 3. Large effusions of blood in the brain or its membranes. 4. Pulmonary apoplexy and hæmato-thorax. 5. The sudden bursting of visceral abscesses. 6. Ulcers of the stomach, duodenum, or other parts of the alimentary canal. 7. Extra-uterine fœtation, peri- and retro-uterine hæmatocele, apoplexy of the ovary, rupture of the uterus. 8. Rupture of the urinary or gall-bladder, or of some other viscus, from accidental violence. 9. Cholera and some forms of zymotic diseases.

* Quoted by Woodman and Tidy, "For. Med." p. 636.

10. Large draughts of cold water when heated. 11. Mental emotions (fear, grief, joy). 12. Foreign bodies accidentally swallowed, and obstructing the glottis.

Ferrario and Sormoni found the sudden deaths in Milan to be distributed as follows:—Head (apoplexy, cerebral concussion, vertigo, and coma), 879, or about 4 in 5. Heart (angina pectoris, aneurism, and hæmorrhage), 150, or about 1 in 7. Lungs (asphyxia, suffocative catarrh, and pulmonary apoplexy), 14, or about 1 in 75. Difficult labours, 5 ; total 1048.

The relative frequency of the different forms of sudden death, classified according to their proximate causes, must, however, be understood to differ at different periods of life. The above proportions are obviously those that obtain chiefly among adults ; for sudden deaths in infancy and childhood, if classed according to their causes, would reverse the order just stated. By far the most frequent cause of death in infancy and childhood is to be found in the lungs, and the least common in the brain. The diseases of the lungs which give rise to sudden or speedy death in infants and young children are spasmodic croup or laryngismus stridulus, to which Dr. West attributes three out of four of the sudden deaths of children under one year, imperfect expansion of the lungs at birth (atelectasis pulmonum), sudden collapse of the lung, consolidation from pneumonia, and sudden serous effusion into the pleura, to which ought to be added a disease not mentioned in the paper now referred to—pulmonary apoplexy. A not uncommon cause of sudden death among the children of the poor is suffocation, as a consequence of drinking hot water from the spout of the kettle. Next to diseases of the lungs, sudden death by exhaustion from insufficient food, or chronic diarrhœa, is most common ; while fatal disorders of the brain are very rare among the causes of sudden death in infancy and childhood.* Of the sudden deaths entered in the tables of the Registrar-General upwards of one-third occur in infancy.

SURVIVORSHIP.

When two or more persons die by the same accident, a question may arise as to which died first ; for in certain cases the succes-

* See a Lecture by Dr. West on Sudden Death in Infancy and Childhood in the *Medical Times and Gazette*, Nov. 26, 1859.

sion to property would be secured on proof of survivorship even for an instant.

Little has yet been done towards establishing general principles applicable to this class of inquiries, chiefly from want of the requisite materials. Some of the more accurate results which have been attained will be found stated under the following heads:—

I. OF THE PROBABILITIES AFFORDED BY AGE AND SEX, IRRESPECTIVE OF THE MODE OF DEATH.

II. OF THE DEGREE IN WHICH SUCH PROBABILITIES ARE AFFECTED BY THE MODE OF DEATH.

I. OF THE PROBABILITIES AFFORDED BY AGE AND SEX.

Age.—As the body attains its full growth and strength at about 27 years of age, or from 25 to 30, and healthy persons continue strong and vigorous up to about 50, there will be no sufficient ground for inferring survivorship in the case of adults of the same sex whose ages range between 25 and 45, or even between 20 and 50, provided the form of death be one in which mere strength and power of endurance is concerned. Before and after the ages specified these will be less; but still within the limits of puberty and old age (say 15 and 60 years) the difference will probably be inconsiderable. The probability of survivorship in the case of a middle-aged adult perishing with one under puberty or above 60, will be in favour of the adult. In the case of one under 15 and one above 60 perishing together, the French law assumes that the former survived: when both are under 15, that the elder outlived the younger. According to the civil law of England, if parent and child perish by a common death, the child is presumed to have survived if above, and to have died first if under, puberty.

In the case of a mother and child both dying in childbed, without assistance, the presumption is that the mother survived; for there is a chance of still birth, and a further probability that the child, if born alive, would die before the mother could render it the assistance necessary. A large child would be still more likely to perish first, for, as elsewhere stated, still-born children greatly exceed in size and weight those born alive. If the child's body could be examined, the presumption might be strengthened by the marks of a difficult labour, or the absence of the signs of respiration. Legal decisions, however, have not always been in conformity with the principle here laid down.

Sex.—If a male and female perish by a common accident in which strength and courage give the best chance of safety, it may be inferred that the male, being the stronger, is the survivor. But females, being subject to prolonged faintings from fright, may be, by that very circumstance, incapacitated from those struggles which in so many forms of death may be presumed to increase danger. When, then, there is safety in exertion, the probability of survivorship will be with the male; when in passive endurance or insensibility, with the female.

II. OF THE DEGREE IN WHICH THE FOREGOING PROBABILITIES ARE AFFECTED BY THE MODE OF DEATH.

Under this head some common modes of death will be specified, and an attempt will be made to establish some general principles with respect to them, assuming, as before, that the parties about whom the question is raised are placed, as nearly as may be, in the same circumstances.

Asphyxia.—Women consume less oxygen than men; hence the same quantity of air will last them for a longer time; and of adult males and females perishing together by asphyxia, the females may be presumed to have survived. In poisoning by the oxides of carbon, the chances of survivorship are with the female. This statement rests on the authority of a large number of facts. In 19 out of 360 cases of poisoning by charcoal fumes which took place in Paris during 1834 and 1835, a man and woman were exposed to these gases together: of these, three only were saved, and these were females. In solitary cases of the same form of death the result is also favourable to the female; for 18 out of 73 females were restored, and only 19 out of 83 males, so that the chances for the female and male respectively are nearly as 15 and 14 (instead of 5 and 4 as Devergie represents it). Single cases are in conformity with this result. Thus, in a case quoted by Beck from the *Transylvania Journal* a man and his wife were exposed in a small room to the gas from live coals. The man was found dead and rigid, but the woman was still breathing, and recovered. Again, in a case reported by M. Sardaillon, a man, his wife, and their child aged seven years, were asphyxiated in a porter's lodge. The child died, the father was very ill, and with difficulty restored to life, while the wife was able to call for help and to assist both husband and child. In these cases we must take into account the position the parties occupied in the room, whether on the bed or floor, near to or remote from an open window, &c.

Drowning.—There are many complicated considerations connected with this mode of death. In shipwrecks men are more likely to be in a favourable situation for saving themselves, as they are more on deck, less encumbered by clothing, more likely to be able to swim, or to cling to floating portions of the wreck. When the comparison is between men similarly exposed and capable of the same exertion, we may have to inquire whether one was more exposed to cold by having the body half immersed, while the other was more under water. Search should also be made for severe injuries which may have prevented the swimmer from using his strength, or may have otherwise proved fatal. Apoplexy is stated by Devergie to be sooner fatal than asphyxia, while in syncope there is the best chance of recovery.

Suffocation.—In all cases of suffocation depending upon an insufficient quantity of air, or upon air rendered partially unfit for respiration, it may be presumed that those who require least air live the longest—women longer than men, children than adults. In suffocation from the falling of houses or earth, or by mechanical means in general, the stronger may be presumed to survive the weaker—*e.g.*, men survive women; and adults, children and old persons.

Cold.—As young children bear cold worse than adults, the probability of survivorship in exposure to the same degree of cold is in favour of the latter. Men bear cold better than women, adults better than the aged. It is necessary also to take into account the clothing of the exposed persons and their state of health. Spirituous liquors in excess increase the effect of cold.

Heat.—The young and old, as they suffer more from cold, so do they bear heat better. The relative tolerance of heat of the two sexes is not well ascertained. Foderé relates the case of an

Englishman and his daughter, aged 7 years, who, in the year 1814, crossed the desert of Syria to the Persian Gulf. Both rode on camels, and were placed in precisely similar circumstances, but the father died, while the child arrived safe at its journey's end. This result might, however, be explained by the greater exertion which the parent would have to make.

Hunger and thirst.—Those who have not reached their full growth require more nourishment than adults, and adults more than aged persons. The aged, then, if healthy and robust, may be presumed to survive both, and the adult to live longer than the child. Corpulent persons are thought to bear hunger better than the spare. In death from starvation, free access to water greatly lengthens life. Those who use most exertion suffer earliest in this as in the foregoing modes of death; while those who possess most passive endurance may be expected to live the longest.

Such are some of the forms of death in which the circumstances of the several victims are likely to be so similar as to admit of the application of general rules. In other modes of death, and in these under certain circumstances, there may be no points admitting of strict comparison, and many things which may exercise a marked influence on the result will have to be taken into account, The reader will find several such cases quoted in Beck's "Medical Jurisprudence"; but as they throw little light upon the general question, and establish no fixed principles, they are not quoted here.

It has been suggested that a distinct enactment would be preferable to the custom of deciding each case on its own merits. Such an enactment, extending to that large class of cases in which the circumstances of the death are imperfectly known, and in which, in the nature of things, it is impossible to come to a correct decision, is certainly much to be desired.

CHAPTER II.

DROWNING—HANGING—STRANGULATION—SUFFOCATION.

THESE modes of death are brought together in the the same chapter, as they all involve asphyxia, or death beginning at the lungs.

DEATH BY DROWNING.

The medico-legal importance of this subject may be inferred from the fact that, in 1893, 3412 deaths were caused by drowning, of which 2766 occurred in males and 646 in females. Of this number, 581 (363 males and 218 females) were ascertained acts of suicide.

Death by drowning is commonly attributed to asphyxia; but it is not always due to that cause. It will be necessary, therefore, to describe the various modes in which a man who has died in the water may have come by his death.

When a man in perfect possession of his faculties falls into the water, he sinks to a greater or less depth, but immediately rises to the surface again; and, if he is a swimmer, makes efforts to save himself, till at length he is reduced to the condition of one who cannot swim at all: with this difference, that he has already exhausted the strength which the other has in reserve for the death struggles which both undergo. These struggles consist of irregular movements of the arms and legs, and grasping of the hands at all objects within reach, whether floating in the water, fixed at the bottom, or growing on the banks. In the course of these irregular movements he rises repeatedly to the surface, tries to breathe, and takes in air and water. The contact of the water with the windpipe causes a cough, by which part of the fluid is rejected, and with it some air from the lungs. This occurs again and again, till the body no longer rises to the surface; water alone is received in the vain efforts to inspire, while forcible involuntary expirations continue to expel air from the chest. At length all these efforts cease, the body sinks to the bottom, and bubbles of air are forced out by the elastic reaction of the walls of the chest. Most of the water entering the mouth finds its way into the stomach, the rest into the lungs; and this residue, mixed with the secretions of the mouth and air-passages, and frothed by the air inspired and expired, forms the foam so constantly met with in persons who have perished in this way.

In these cases we find the characteristic marks of asphyxia, coupled with those due to the medium in which the death takes place. In the case of the swimmer death may take place from exhaustion, with less distinct marks of asphyxia.

But death may take place in the water, and yet be caused neither by asphyxia nor by exhaustion. There may be complete loss of consciousness at the moment of immersion. This may happen from fright, drunkenness, an attack of hysteria, or of catalepsy (of which we have known one instance—G.): and in this case the body falls to the bottom, rises again to a certain height, and sinks without a struggle, death being due to shock or to syncope.

A man may fall or throw himself into the water head foremost, and striking against some solid substance, or even against the water itself, perish by concussion; or falling or being thrown from a height, may strike the water with the chest and pit of the stomach, and die instantly from shock.

Again, cold, excitement, or the first violent struggles may occasion apoplexy, or sudden death from disease of the heart. Such deaths occasionally occur in persons bathing in cold, shallow water.

Death by drowning may also be of a mixed character. A man falls into the water in full possession of all his faculties, which he preserves for a time, till, struck with horror at the death which threatens him, he faints, and thus perishes.

It appears, then, that death by drowning may be due to asphyxia, to exhaustion, to shock, to syncope, and to apoplexy; or partly to asphyxia, partly to one or other of the causes just specified, and these mixed cases are much the most common; while those in which asphyxia and its signs are wholly absent form a small minority, and cases of pure and unmixed asphyxia occupy an intermediate place. Devergie, whose large experience of the drowned has been already alluded to, estimates the cases of unmixed asphyxia as *two in eight* of the whole, the cases in which no trace of asphyxia exist as *one in eight*, and the mixed cases as *five-eighths*.

The appearance in the body of the drowned must necessarily vary with the manner and cause of death.

Where death has been due to asphyxia the post-mortem appearances will be those proper to that mode of death (see p. 307), blended with those due to the medium in which the death happened, and modified by the time the body has remained in the water, as well as by the length of the subsequent exposure to the air.

If in death by asphyxia the examination be made soon after the death and removal from the water, the following appearances may be present :—The face and general surface of the body are pale or slightly livid, with patches of a deeper tint. The expression of the face is generally calm. The tongue is swollen, and closely applied to the teeth, rarely protruded between the closed jaws, and still more rarely wounded and bloody; and there is a frothy foam at the mouth. The air-passages also contain a froth, sometimes tinged with blood; and the trachea and larger bronchial tubes contain water, which penetrates to their most minute ramifications, and may fill the whole of the air-passages. The water occasionally carries with it slime or mud, or fragments of aquatic plants. The lining membrane of the air-passages is sometimes congested; the lungs are distended and œdematous, and exude a sanguinolent frothy liquid when incised. The venæ cavæ and right side of the heart are filled with dark blood, while the left cavities are comparatively empty. The stomach contains water, sometimes in considerable quantity. The intestines have a rosy colour; the liver, spleen, and kidneys are gorged with blood, and the bladder sometimes contains bloody urine. The brain presents the same appearances as in other cases of death by asphyxia. Sand or mud may be found in the hollow of the nails, the fingers are sometimes abraded, and portions of plants growing in the water, or on the banks of the stream, may be found grasped in the hands. Injuries received in falling into the water during the death-struggles, or through the violence of the stream, may also leave their marks upon the body.

In bodies that have remained in the water or been exposed to the air for some time, the pallid or slightly livid hue of the features may be exchanged for a bloated appearance, the large livid spots may show themselves on different parts of the body, as in other cases of death by asphyxia.

In death by shock, syncope, or exhaustion, there is little or no water in the air-passages or stomach; the cavities of the heart and the large vessels are equally distended with blood, or are nearly empty, and the brain and internal viscera are in their natural state.

Death by concussion, asphyxia, apoplexy, or disease of the heart, reveals itself by the usual post-mortem appearances.

In mixed cases, the appearances due to asphyxia are less strongly marked. There is less froth at the mouth, less water and froth in the air-passages and stomach, less congestion of the lungs, heart and great vessels and internal viscera.

WAS DEATH CAUSED BY DROWNING?

In the case of a body found in the water, death may obviously have happened prior to immersion from natural causes, or from some form of violent death, such as hanging or strangulation, which gives rise to the characteristic appearances of asphyxia, so that we have to consider whether the post-mortem appearances alleged to be characteristic of death by drowning might have been occasioned by causes acting before immersion; and whether, in the case of bodies which have remained in the water some time, the appearances usually attributed to the mode of death may not be explained by the circumstances of the immersion itself.

The post-mortem appearances alleged to be due to drowning, and to be characteristic of it, must now be briefly considered.

Of the **external signs** of drowning, those which are first noticed are the flowing of water from the mouth on turning the body face downwards, and the presence of froth at the lips and nostrils. The first sign failed in two cases only out of 26 in which it was carefully looked for by F. Ogston, jun.; and in both these decomposition was far advanced.

Froth at the mouth and nostrils.—This is a sign of death by drowning, but open to all the objections stated on p. 321 in respect of froth in the air-passages. It has, indeed, a close dependence on the existence of froth in the air-passages, but it is always seen most copiously shortly after death. Contrary to the generally accepted belief, that it appears sooner in summer than in winter, owing to its propulsion from the air-passages by development of gas, Ogston states that it appears sooner in winter than in summer. It rapidly disappears when the body is exposed to the air.[*] F. Ogston, jun., considers it a reliable sign when observed soon after the removal of the body from the water. He noticed it at the mouth in 20 per cent. of the cases, and at the nostrils in 12·9 per cent. The red froth sometimes observed is not confined to the drowned, and occurs in bodies advanced in putrefaction.

Condition of the skin—Cutis anserina.—The skin is usually stated to be of great pallor; but frequently over the face and front of the chest it is of a rosy-red colour. In death by drowning, whether in summer or winter, the body exhibits the appearance known as "goose-skin," or cutis anserina. This is caused by the contracted state of the *arrectores pili*, and is chiefly seen on the anterior surface of the extremities. The cutis anserina may, however, be found in death from other causes, and particularly in cases of sudden death with nervous excitement. Taken by itself, its presence does not prove death by drowning, but its absence would be a serious objection, unless other signs were unusually pronounced.

Condition of the penis.—Casper alleges that, in men who have fallen into the water alive and died by drowning, he has almost never failed to find retraction of this organ, while he has not observed it so constantly after any other kind of death. ("Handbook," vol. ii. p. 236.) It is not, however, universal; and Ogston, jun., confirms other medical jurists in finding semi-erection as the more common condition. Thus, in 72 cases semi-erection was present in 58·3 per cent., retraction in 23·6 per cent. and erection in 16·6 per cent.[†]

Excoriations of the fingers are much more often absent than present; but when they exist, may be regarded as a probable

---

* "Lect. on Med. Jurisp.," p. 508.
† Ogston, jun., *Edin. Med. Journal*, April 1882.

though not certain sign. They might be caused previous to forcible immersion, by the rubbing of the fingers against any hard and rough body, and possibly after death in running streams.

Sand or mud in the hollow of the nails also affords a probability of immersion during life, for it implies, like excoriations of the fingers, that the drowning man grasped at the bed or banks. But if the body remained long in the water, mud or sand might be deposited in the nails.

Hands clenched and grasping weeds growing in the stream or on the banks afford the strongest probability of death by drowning.

Of the **internal signs** of drowning, the most important are the condition of the digestive tract and the respiratory tract.

Water in the stomach.—This also affords strong presumption in favour of death by drowning; especially if the water (or other fluid) can be identified with that in which the body was found by its containing leaves of plants growing on the banks or at the bottom. Except in the cases presently to be mentioned, it presupposes acts of deglutition during efforts to breathe. It is, however, possible, though very unlikely, that the water might have been swallowed a very short time before submersion.

The quantity of water depends partly on the number of respiratory efforts made during the act of drowning, and partly on the depth of the water. In animals stunned before immersion, as well as in those prevented from rising to the surface, the stomach contains no water; while in animals free to move it is found to be in proportion to the number of times they rise.

That the depth of the water also influences the quantity found in the stomach is proved by the experiments of Dr. Taylor. The stomach of a cat held two feet below the surface of the Thames contained scarcely any water; that of a cat lowered to the depth of fifty-five feet held a large quantity; while the stomach of a third cat, allowed to rise repeatedly to the surface, held a quantity of water intermediate between the other two. The columnar pressure of the water is therefore of some influence in determining the amount of water in the stomach; and it is probable that when the water is very deep it may force the passage of the œsophagus, even though the animal died previously to submersion. But repeated experiments on animals have shown that, as a rule, water does not enter the stomach after death—not at least until the tissues have been relaxed by putrefaction.*

It is obvious, then, that water in the stomach is not to be taken as conclusive of death by drowning, when the water is of great depth, or the body far advanced in putrefaction. It must also be admitted that the water might have been swallowed just before immersion, and possible, also, though most improbable, that it might, as suggested by Orfila, be maliciously injected after death.

On the other hand, the absence of water from the stomach must not be taken as evidence that the death was not caused by drowning; for it is not present in death by drowning due to causes other than asphyxia, such as shock, syncope, concussion, or apoplexy. The tendency to swallow may also be resisted; or the body may be, in some way or other, prevented from rising to the surface.

Again, water may have entered the stomach, and yet not be found there after death, if the head be allowed to hang down, as was proved by Dr. Taylor's experiments. Again, by long exposure after removal from the water, the fluid in the stomach may transude through its coats, and disappear.

Froth, water, mud, or sand in the air-passages.—Mucous froth.—From the experiments of Piorry and Orfila on animals, the presence of mucous froth in the air-passages was inferred to be due to the body rising repeatedly to the surface for air. In animals kept entirely under water no froth was found; and it was also absent when the body remained in the water a long time, or was subject to long exposure after its removal; as also when the head was placed downwards. But Casper, as the result

* The experiments of Liman (Casper's "Handbuch," vol. ii. p. 747, 5th edition) seem to throw considerable doubt on the value of the presence of water in the stomach as a sign of submersion during life. His experiments consisted in submerging the dead bodies of children in an artificial morass compounded of water and easily recognisable material. The bodies were placed in this, some with the face upwards, some quite submerged, and then taken out after a day or two by the head or feet, or in no definite manner. In sixteen experiments the material was found in the stomach seven times, and in the œsophagus, pharynx, and trachea fourteen times. Neither the degree of putrefaction nor the length of time during which the bodies were allowed to lie in the morass appeared to influence the result; nor did it matter whether the bodies were drawn out by the head or heels. He concludes from his experiments that the occurrence of water in the stomach or air-passages may be purely a post-mortem accident. Hoffmann, however, states that in his experiments water was never found in the smaller bronchial tubes, and only a slight obstruction, as by mucus, in the œsophagus or bronchial tubes was sufficient to prevent the entrance of water. ("Lehrbuch der gerichtlich. Med.," 1881, p. 518.)

of numerous observations, affirms that these experiments are not applicable to the human subject. He found froth in the trachea equally in those who could and those who could not have risen to the surface. The value of this evidence of death by drowning is also impaired by the fact that mucous froth exists not only in the several forms of death by asphyxia, but in death by apoplexy, or epilepsy, and in catarrhal and other affections of the lungs.

Ogston,[*] however, states that the froth of drowning can be distinguished from frothy mucus due to other causes by its whitish, rarely sanguinolent appearance, forming a kind of lather composed of minute bubbles, with a watery envelope easily ruptured.

Condition of the lungs.—On opening the chest the lungs bulge considerably, and are often, in fact, what may be called " balloon " lungs. That water generally enters the lungs in death by drowning has been abundantly proved by experiments on animals, and by cases in the human subject in which sand and mud and leaves of plants have entered the air-passages. By drowning rats in chalk and water, with free access to the air, I have never failed to obtain effervescence by means of acids in every part of the lungs (G.).

But the value of this sign is impaired by the fact that water may enter the lungs of those who have been thrown in after death. Orfila and Piorry found that the quantity which thus gained admission varies according to the position of the body, being large when it remained upright, less when horizontal.

But water is not always present in the lungs in death by drowning; for, as in the case of the stomach, if the head is placed downwards the water flows out. Long exposure, too, will cause it to transude and be lost. The suggestion that water may be *injected* after death may be treated as a fanciful refinement.

From this examination of the signs of death by drowning it appears that there is no one sign on which entire reliance can be placed; but when several signs coincide, the probability is greatly strengthened. Some authors—Orfila among the number—have thought that the question, Was death due to drowning? admits of no decision; but from this opinion Devergie and Casper very properly dissent.

It should also be borne in mind that the most characteristic

* " Lect. on Med. Jurisp.," p. 508.

appearances are not permanent. In winter they may continue after the body has lain from fifteen to eighteen days in the water, but in summer they may disappear as early as the third day. Under exposure to the air they also rapidly pass away, and in the height of summer a few hours may suffice to dissipate them. Advanced putrefaction destroys all the signs of death by drowning.

The time that the body has remained in the water will be determined approximately by the signs laid down at p. 300.

The evidence derived from the signs of death by drowning admits of being confirmed or invalidated by the condition of the body in other respects, especially by the presence or absence of

Marks of violence on the drowned.—With regard to injuries on the bodies of persons found in the water, three questions arise :

1. Were they inflicted during life ?   2. If so, are they such as to account for death before submersion ?   3. Were they accidental, suicidal, or homicidal ?

The first and third questions are fully discussed under the head of " Wounds." The immersion of the body in water will influence the decision of these questions only in so far as the injuries are thereby altered in appearance.

Are the injuries such as to account for death from submersion ?—There are five ways in which a body taken from the water may come to exhibit marks of violence : 1. A man may be murdered (by poison or other means), and thrown into the water dead ; 2. He may receive severe injuries from the hands of others or himself, and may then be thrown (or throw himself) into the water while still alive. If the injuries are in the shape of bruises, they may have been caused—3. By the death struggles ; 4. By some obstacle against which the body is borne ; 5. In the very act of falling into the water.

1. In a man who has been murdered and thrown into the water dead, we should expect to find all the signs of death by drowning absent, with the exception of such as may have been caused by uncommon depth of water or advanced putrefaction.

2. On the supposition that a man found in the water had first been severely injured and then thrown in alive, we might expect to find signs of drowning proportioned in number and distinctness to the strength still left after the violence inflicted.

3. The bruises caused by the struggles of the drowning man would not be so severe or extensive as to endanger life.

4. The bruises caused by fixed obstacles, against which the body might be borne by a running stream, would not be strongly marked. It is not likely that such severe injuries as dislocations or fractures could originate in this way, unless the obstacle were in motion—*e.g.*, a water-wheel, screw, or paddle.

5. A person who falls or throws himself from a height upon a hard bank or pier of a bridge may not only be severely bruised, but sustain such injuries as fractures of the skull or limbs, and extensive lacerated wounds.

Dislocation of the limbs is a possible consequence of falling from a great height. Many years since, as stated by Dr. Gordon Smith, a man who used to jump from the parapet of London Bridge into the Thames for a wager, and had previously performed the feat with impunity, sank and was drowned. Both arms were found dislocated, in consequence, it is thought, of his having fallen with them stretched out, instead of close to his sides, as was his wont.

Two cases are also recorded (South's edition of Chelius's "Surgery," vol. i. p. 532), the one of fracture of the body and arch of the fourth cervical vertebra, and the other of fracture of the body of the fifth vertebra, caused by jumping into the water. The deaths were attributed to a sudden retraction of the head to avert collision with the bottom.

We should therefore ascertain whether the drowned man fell from a height; whether the water is a rapid stream, and whether the body was found near obstacles fixed or in motion; and if there are no such causes as these to account for the injuries sustained, we may fairly trace them to some cause preceding the immersion. In bodies found in shallow, still water, marks of violence afford a strong presumption of homicide.

Assuming death to have been due to drowning, the question arises:

Was the drowning the result of accident, suicide, or homicide?—This question is exceedingly difficult to answer; for if there are no marks of violence on the body, it is not possible to say whether the man fell in, or jumped in, or was pushed in; and in respect of bodies found in running streams, it may not be possible to ascertain at what point they entered the water.

Nor, if we find the hands of the drowned man grasping leaves or grass, showing that he had struggled hard while in the water, can we affirm that he was thrown or pushed in by others.

Nor again, does the fact of a man being drowned in a shallow stream of water exclude the idea of homicide ; for if a strong man were to hold the head of a weak or infirm one in a basin of water, he might drown him as effectually as in a deep stream. On the other hand, cases of suicidal drowning in shallow water, or in narrow spaces, such as small house-cisterns, are on record.

It is evident, from what has been stated, that in the absence of marks of violence we have no means of determining whether the drowning was due to accident, suicide, or homicide ; and that such marks, to throw any light upon the question, must be such as could not have been inflicted by the drowned man himself prior to immersion, or by the accidental striking of the body against an obstacle in entering the water or during the death struggle.

There is one case which at first sight would seem conclusive of homicide—namely, where a body is found in the water tied hand and foot. Dr Smith, however, relates the following case :—In July 1816, the body of a gauging-instrument maker, who had been missing for some days, was discovered floating down the Thames. His wrists were found tied together, and made fast to his knees, which were also secured to each other. He had been deranged for two years. The cord with which he had tied himself was recognised as that with which he used to raise himself in bed. He was a good swimmer, and probably adopted this means of disabling himself. The verdict was " Found drowned." Two similar cases are on record, one by Foderé, in which the hands and fingers were tied together with a silk riband in numerous folds ; and another in which the feet, wrists, and neck were tied. Foderé in the one case, and the medical examiners (Marc, Guichard, &c.) in the other, gave their opinion in favour of suicide. In such cases as these it would be necessary to determine whether the knots or folds could have been made with the teeth, or by any movements of the hands or limbs.

Resuscitation from drowning.—The insensibility which supervenes on asphyxia brought about by obstruction of the respiration is not synonymous with death for though all spontaneous respiratory movements have ceased, resuscitation is possible so long as the heart continues to beat.

As, then, in such cases of obstructed respiration, the heart may continue to beat for several minutes after every respiratory movement has ceased, all hope of resuscitation need not be abandoned though no respiratory movements can be perceived. But in asphyxia produced by drowning, even though the heart may continue to beat, resuscitation can rarely be brought about after complete submersion lasting for so short a period as two minutes, or even less than this. Thus the longest time the Navarino sponge-divers can remain under water is 76 seconds; though in 1882 a woman who was exhibiting in London remained under water for 2½ to 3 minutes at a time. The cause of the difficulty of resuscitation after submersion is the entrance of water into the lungs, which renders them incapable of collapsing and aërating the blood by the methods resorted to. Many cases of resuscitation after submersion for a longer period are on record. Some of these may be discarded as untrustworthy, and ascribed to exaggeration of time by anxious onlookers. Others, however, may be referred to the supervention of syncope at the moment of immersion, in consequence of which the aspiration of water into the lungs has not occurred to any extent; and some perhaps to the success attending the first efforts made to free the lungs from water.

In the treatment of the drowned, or of asphyxia in general, recourse must be had to artificial respiration. But the special circumstances of drowning require that means be used to counteract the great loss of heat which occurs even in the greatest summer temperature, and also precautions to remove from the air-passages the accumulated mucus and fluids which obstruct them.

The following rules for the treatment of the drowned are in accordance with the method of Dr. Henry Silvester, which has now, by general consent, taken the place of that recommended by Dr. Marshall Hall :—Send immediately for blankets and dry clothing, but treat the patient instantly on the spot, in the open air. First place the body, for a few seconds, with the face downwards, the head lower than the feet, the mouth open, and the tongue drawn forward; then turn the body on the back, place it on an inclined surface, raise the shoulders and support them, and fix the feet. Now grasp the arms at the elbows, draw them above the head, and keep them on the stretch for two seconds; then reverse the movement for the same length of time, pressing the arms firmly against the sides of the chest. Repeat this twofold movement fifteen times in the minute, till a spontaneous effort at respiration occurs. Then remit the movements, and proceed to promote the circulation and restore warmth by firm friction and pressure directed upwards, by hot flannels, hot bottles, bladders of hot water, or heated bricks; or borrow warm clothing from the bystanders. Respiration may be promoted by smelling salts, tickling the throat with a feather, and by the alternate dash of cold and warm water on the face and chest. When the respiration is restored, warm brandy and water, wine and water, tea or coffee, may be given; and the patient, being put to bed, should be allowed to sleep. Our efforts to restore life should be persevered in for three or four hours, or till some certain sign of death has shown itself.

Howard's* method of artificial respiration.—Howard recommends that the accumulated fluids should first be got rid of by placing the body in a prone position, with a roll of clothing beneath the stomach, and pressing on the spine till this is effected. The body is then laid supine with a roll of clothing in the hollow of the back, so as to render the epigastrium prominent. The arms are drawn upwards, held by the hand of an assistant, whose other hand is employed in keeping the tongue drawn out at the corner of the mouth with a cloth. The operator then kneels astride or at the side of the patient, places his hands on the short ribs, then pivoting himself on his knees, throws the weight of his body forward on the hands, which at the same time squeeze the chest walls. He then lets go suddenly, so as to allow an inspiration, and this alternate compression and relaxation is to be carried out about fifteen times per minute.

DEATH BY HANGING.

In the year 1892, 671 persons perished by hanging in England, of whom 532 were males and 139 females. All these deaths were ascertained suicidal acts.

As asphyxia is a cause of death common to hanging, strangulation, and suffocation, a few general observations will be made on these modes of death before proceeding to examine them separately.

* The Direct Method of Artificial Respiration : *Trans. Amer. Med. Assoc.,* vol. xxii. 1871.

Though it is usual to say of death from these three causes that it is due to suffocation, this term has in medico-legal language a distinct meaning of its own. It means death caused by some impediment to the respiration which does not act by compressing the larynx or trachea. Thus, a man is said to be suffocated if his mouth and nostrils are closed, or if he is prevented from breathing by pressure on the chest or abdomen. Certain noxious gases, too, are said to kill by suffocation. In hanging, strangulation, and throttling, death is caused by pressure exercised on the air-tube and throat.

The most simple cause of death is throttling, or direct pressure on the trachea with the fingers. Here the cause is obvious; it is the same as in many cases of drowning; the same as in suffocation—viz., asphyxia (apnœa). Death takes place from the mechanical hindrance to respiration. But the cause of death is not so clear when the entire circumference of the neck is subject to pressure; for then not only the larynx or trachea, but the blood-vessels may be pressed upon. In some instances both air-tubes and blood-vessels are implicated; in others the air-tubes suffer compression and the vessels escape; in others, again, the air-tubes escape and the vessels sustain the pressure. The respiration and circulation are most completely impeded when a cord is fixed round the lower part of the neck, so as to embrace the trachea and the large vessels at their entrance into and exit from the chest; or when it is applied, or drawn by the weight of the body, beneath the lower jaw. Both functions are less interfered with when the cord is fixed directly over the larynx, as the projections of the os hyoides and thyroid cartilage afford some protection to the windpipe and blood-vessels.

This variation in the position of the ligature, and in the consequent pressure on the organs of respiration and circulation respectively, explains the difference in the time required to destroy life in all those cases in which death does not take place instantaneously from shock or injury to the spinal cord; and the simultaneous compression of the air-tube and blood-vessels gives rise to the question, whether the pressure on the air-tube or on the blood-vessels is the immediate cause of death. In other words, is death caused by asphyxia or by coma?

It was formerly the general belief that death was due to coma; and this opinion was not unreasonable, for it is well known that mere pressure with the fingers on the carotid artery will cause sleep, by checking the supply of blood to the brain, and that apoplexy is often brought on, in persons predisposed, by the pressure of a cravat impeding the return of blood through the veins. That coma, therefore, may be brought about by pressure on the large blood-vessels is not to be doubted, but the question still recurs—in those cases of suspension or strangulation in which the air-tube and blood-vessels are simultaneously compressed, which of the two pressures causes death ? Both causes doubtless contribute to the fatal result, but the stoppage of the respiration is certainly the essential cause; for death by asphyxia would be much more speedily and certainly induced by a complete or partial stoppage of the breathing, than fatal coma by the complete or partial arrest of the circulation. But an appeal may be made to actual experiment for the decision of this question. A dog was suspended by the neck with a cord, an opening having been made in the trachea below the place where the cord was applied. After hanging about three-quarters of an hour, during which time the circulation and breathing went on as usual, the animal was cut down, and did not appear to have suffered much. The cord was then shifted below the opening, so as to stop the ingress of air into the lungs; and the animal being again suspended, was in a few minutes quite dead. In this experiment the compression was less that it would be in many cases of death by hanging in the human subject, in which the violence employed, the height of the fall, and the weight of the body combine to tighten the cord, and thus exercise the strongest pressure on the vessels as well as on the air-tube.

A similar operation has been performed on the human subject.[*]

"A man of the name of Gordon was executed at Tyburn in April 1733. Mr. Chovet having by frequent experiments on dogs discovered that opening the windpipe would prevent the fatal consequences of the halter, undertook to save Gordon, and accordingly made an incision in his windpipe, the effect of which was, that when Gordon stopped his mouth, nostrils, and ears for some time, air enough came through the opening to allow of the continuance of life. When hanged, he was observed to be alive after all the rest were dead; and when he had hung three-

_____

[*] Smith's "Forensic Medicine," Appendix, p. 561.

quarters of an hour, being carried to a house in the Tyburn road, he opened his mouth several times and groaned, and a vein being opened he bled freely." But these were the only signs of life. Smith attributed the want of success to the great weight of the man, coupled perhaps with the insufficiency of the opening into the trachea.

It appears, then, that when the windpipe and the large blood-vessels suffer compression, death may be attributed to asphyxia: that when the respiration is free, or but slightly affected, pressure on the vessels may cause death by coma, but more slowly; and that when respiration and circulation are both impeded, both may contribute to the fatal result, though the hindrance to the respiration is the more efficient.

It has been suggested that the immediate cause of death in hanging and strangulation is pressure on the nerves which subserve the function of respiration; but as such pressure does not prove fatal till the lapse of many hours, this explanation must be rejected.

Having now examined the questions common to death by hanging and by strangulation, the subject of death by hanging may be resumed.

Death takes place very suddenly in certain cases of suspension, as in some cases of drowning, either from shock or syncope, or from injury to the spinal cord by luxation of the cervical vertebræ, fracture of the odontoid process, or rupture of the intervertebral substance, these injuries to the spine being caused either by the fall of the body from a height, or by a rotatory motion given to the body at the moment of the fall.

Death by hanging takes place, then, in different ways and at different intervals of time. The quicker deaths may be traced to injury of the spinal cord above the origin of the nerves of respiration, and, more rarely, to syncope. Next in rapidity is death from asphyxia, and the least rapid that by coma.

We are not without information as to the sensations that accompany death by hanging. Suicides saved from death, and philosophers who have instituted experiments on themselves, have both contributed something to our knowledge. It appears that these sensations are not always the same; and the difference probably depends on the various degrees in which the windpipe and blood-vessels are compressed. Some have retained no recollection of what happened ; others were conscious of sudden loss of sense and motion ; in others a deep sleep was ushered in by flashes of light, by a bluish flame, by brilliant circles of colours, or by more definite ocular illusions, accompanied by hissing or singing in the ears. In other instances the sensations are stated to have been extremely pleasurable, though of short duration. These sensations resemble those that are caused by disordered cerebral circulation, and those that usher in the fits in some cases of epilepsy. But it is only in cases of suicide that these pleasurable sensations manifest themselves. In homicidal cases, especially when much violence is used, there are signs of great suffering.

Appearances after death.—The appearances found after death by hanging are not uniform or constant, and there is no single sign invariably present diagnostic of death by hanging. Indication of suspension, but not necessarily of death by such means, is the mark of the cord on the neck, usually lying above the hyoid bone, obliquely upwards behind the ears, and losing itself in the occiput. The mark varies, however, in position and character according to the mode of suspension and the nature of the material of which the cord is made (see p. 332). The subcutaneous tissues beneath the mark is compressed or silvery.

Occasionally minute extravasations are seen in the deeper layers of the skin. The middle and internal coats of the carotid may be lacerated, and where the momentum has been great, rupture of the cervical muscles, of the thyro-hyoid ligaments, fracture of the larynx, fracture or dislocation of the cervical vertebræ, with injury to the medulla and effusion into the spinal canal, may be found.

The face is sometimes, but not commonly, distorted and expressive of suffering. Usually it is placid and pale, though after long suspension it may become livid. The eyes are sometimes very prominent, and the pupils are dilated. Frothy mucus may be found at the mouth and nostrils. The tongue is pressed against the teeth and indented, or it may be clenched between the jaws. The base of the tongue is injected. The hands are often tightly clenched, the nails being driven into the palms. Erection or semi-erection of the penis in men, with expulsion of semen or prostatic fluid, and vascular turgescence of the genitals in females, with sanguinolent effusion, are frequently observed ; an expulsion of the contents of the bladder and rectum is also common.

The internal appearances are those of asphyxia (see p. 307), or of asphyxia with marked cerebral congestion. The condition of the brain varies; congestion is sometimes well marked, at other times not noticeable. Cerebral hæmorrhage is extremely rare. In some cases intense congestion of the mucous membrane of the stomach, simulating irritant poisoning, has been found. Where death has resulted from shock or direct injury to the medulla, the signs of asphyxia will be wanting.

Two principal medico-legal questions arise in regard to persons found hanged: **Did the suspension take place during life, or after death?** and **was the hanging accidental, suicidal, or homicidal?**

Did the suspension take place during life, or after death?

The points most worthy of attention as bearing on the solution of this question are: **The mark of the cord; the appearance of the countenance; the position and state of the tongue; the condition of the genital organs;** and **the expulsion of the fæces.**

Mark of the cord.—The appearances on the neck due to suspension during life are not uniform. In homicidal cases the neck sustains great injury, the skin is bruised, and the subjacent parts torn; but in judicial and suicidal hanging much less injury is done both to the skin and to the deeper-seated parts.

In those cases (both judicial and suicidal) in which the position of the cord is mainly determined by the weight of the body, it follows pretty closely the line of the jaw-bone, and there may be an oblique indented mark, of the colour of a recent bruise, on the fore part of the neck, and yellowish-brown, as if from a singe, towards the angle of the jaw. The bruise may correspond with the whole breadth of the ligature; or there may be a deep groove, bordered by two discoloured lines. The mark varies with the size and texture of the cord, being less distinct when a soft material, such as a handkerchief, is used, than when a hard ligature, such as a rope, is employed. When the material is hard and resisting, the number of times that the ligature has been passed round the neck, and the material of which it consists, are clearly displayed. But in many cases of judicial and suicidal hanging the mark of the rope consists at first of a simple depression without any change of colour, oblique if due to the weight of the body, horizontal if firmly fixed round the neck. After the lapse of several hours, the rope-mark assumes a light-brownish tint, and if an incision be made into the skin, the cellular tissue is found strongly compressed, so as to form a shining white band. Occasionally injection of the skin at the bottom of the groove is found, or even minute ecchymoses of the *cutis vera* (Neyding and Bremme). Sometimes the pressure is lessened by the beard, or it is not equal on the two sides, or the back of the neck escapes. The face, as will be presently more fully stated, is at first pale and its expression natural, and it is not till several hours have elapsed that it grows livid, and still longer before it wears a bloated appearance.

In a case of judicial hanging, in which the cord was removed soon after the body had been cut down, we observed merely a depressed circle on the fore part of the neck, and a slight excoriation, with a burnt appearance, over the angle of the jaw. In a case of suicidal hanging with a small rope tied firmly round the neck, but removed without delay, there was a white depressed line, deeper at the back of the neck than in front, and assuming a dusky hue after several hours. The strands of the rope were distinctly marked, but there was no ecchymosis on any part of the neck. In another case of suicidal hanging a hard depressed chocolate-coloured band completely surrounded the neck, and corresponded to the rope of coir which had been used (G.).

In cases, then, of hanging during life, the cord does not always produce the same appearances. Iu some cases there is a well-marked bruise or ecchymosis, in others a pale indentation and a condensed state of the subcutaneous tissues resembling old parchment; in others, again, a hard chocolate-coloured groove; and these marks, limited to the fore part of the neck, may be combined at the angle of the jaw with a singed appearance. The cuticle may also be abraded here and there.

Can the appearances occasioned by the cord during life be produced after death?—This question has been answered in the affirmative. In the chapter on Wounds and Mechanical Injuries it will be shown that bruises may be produced some time after life is extinct; and that which is true of bruises in general will of course hold good with respect to this particular form of bruise. Accordingly, Orfila proved, by experiments on the dead body, that up to eighteen hours after death precisely the same appearances may be produced as in suspension during life;

Devergie has produced the parchment-like condition of the skin and subjacent cellular tissue, as well as the livid appearance bounding the depression; and Casper sums up the results of a long series of experiments by the remarkable statement, "that any ligature with which any body may be suspended or strangled, not only within a few hours, but even days after death, especially if the body be forcibly pulled downwards, may produce a mark precisely similar to that which is observed in most of those hanged while alive;" and he adds that he has been convinced by his experiments that the mark of the cord is a purely cadaveric phenomenon.

But for these confident statements of Casper, based upon several

FIG. 40.

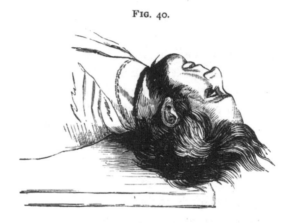

experiments and large experience, I should have attached some value to the depressed chocolate-coloured line which I encountered in one case of suicide, accompanied by so condensed a condition of skin that, when cut, it resembled closely the toughest brawn. The appearance of the neck is well shown in the engraving (Fig. 40) from a photograph, which also displays the results of an experiment made with the cord used in the suspension, fastened tightly round the neck within an hour of the death, and left for about twenty hours. The result was a slightly depressed mark the size of the cord, showing the projecting strands in white depressions, on a faint rose-coloured ground. This mark did not deepen in colour by exposure. The deep indigo blue colour of the ears was very remarkable, though the man had a swarthy complexion.

The suicide had attached a neckerchief to a hook, and passed through the loop the small rope of coir by which he hanged himself. He had mounted a table, which he kicked from under him. His feet nearly touched the floor of the cell (Fig. 41) (G.).

But even in cases in which the mark of the cord is indistinct and not in itself conclusive, the state of the parts beneath the skin may enable us to speak with confidence. A considerable effusion of blood, a rupture of the trachea, a separation of its cartilages, a dislocation of the spine, a division of the coats of the vessels, all of them evidence of great violence, would furnish a strong probability of suspension during life, or of suspension after forcible strangulation.

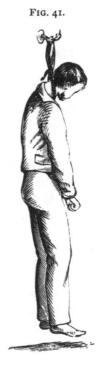

FIG. 41.

The face.—In death by hanging, whether judicial or suicidal, the face is usually pale and its expression natural, though sometimes distorted and expressive of suffering. But the pallor is followed after a few hours by a livid hue of the lips, eyelids, ears, and face generally ; and, after a still longer interval, by a marked congestion of the face. There is nothing in the expression or colour to show whether suspension took place during life or after death, but if the vessels of the head and face are found highly congested in a body recently cut down, there is a probability of suspension during life ; for suspension after death, though it might produce discoloration of the neck, could not cause turgescence of the vessels of the head and face.

Position and state of the tongue.—The same injected and swollen state of the base of the tongue, with or without protrusion, which occurs in other forms of death by asphyxia, occurs also in death by hanging, and affords a strong probability of suspension during life.

State of the genital organs.—The genital organs of both sexes are affected in death by hanging. In the female, redness of the labia and discharge of blood have been noted ; and in the male a more or less complete state of erection of the penis, with discharge of urine, mucus, or prostatic fluid, is present in at least one case in three. There may also be discharge from the urethra without erection. But these appearances in the genital organs, when they do occur, are not characteristic of death by hanging or strangulation, for they have been seen in other forms of violent and sudden death, as in fatal gun-shot wounds of the brain and of the large vessels, and in poisoning by prussic acid.

This sign, then, when present, is very important; for it is strictly vital, and affords a sure proof of violent and sudden death, and, if combined with characteristic external signs and internal appearances, of death by hanging. On the other hand, erection and emission may be absent, and yet death may have been due to this cause.

Expulsion of the fæces. — This happens in about one-fourth of the cases of death by hanging, but as it also occurs in other forms of sudden or violent death, it needs to be confirmed by characteristic appearances, external and internal.

Was the hanging accidental, suicidal, or homicidal? —Accidental hanging is very rare. One case is given by Gordon Smith. It was that of a girl who was swinging in a brewhouse, near a rope used for drawing up slaughtered sheep. Her head got through a noose of this second rope, by which she was pulled out of the swing and kept suspended till she died. Dr. Taylor also relates a case communicated to him by one of his pupils :—A boy, ten years old, fastened a piece of plaid gown to a loop in a cord suspended from a beam, and in the act of swinging, raised and turned himself, when the loop of rope caught him under the chin, and suspended him till life was extinct. A playmate witnessed the occurrence.

Setting aside a few such cases, which can create no difficulty, the question under consideration is narrowed to this : Was the hanging suicidal or homicidal? The figures of the Registrar-General show that the probability is always strongly in favour of suicide; and, for obvious reasons, hanging is a mode of death a murderer is not likely to select. It presupposes a great disproportion of strength between him and his victim, or a combination of two or more persons against one. The solitary ascertained case of homicide in the five years 1852 to 1856 was committed on a young child.

There would be nothing in the appearance of the body itself, beyond the marks of a severe struggle, to distinguish the homicidal from the suicidal act; but if a man were found suspended at a height from the ground which he could not by any possibility have reached, and with no object near on which he could have mounted, we must conclude that he was suspended by another.

It was once thought that a man found with the feet, or some part of the body, touching the ground, was more likely to have been hanged by another than by himself; but this has been shown to be an error, for undoubted suicides have been found with the feet touching the ground in a sitting or half-sitting posture, and even with the knees bent and raised above the ground, or in such postures that death must have been caused by leaning forcibly forward and so compressing the windpipe.*

As in most of these cases the cord would not be drawn by the weight of the body into the usual oblique position, such cases would differ from cases of strangulation only in the mark being less distinct, and embracing a smaller portion of the neck.

The marks of violent struggles on the clothes or person of the deceased would justify a suspicion of homicide; but as severe and extensive injuries have been known to be produced by a suicide, and slighter injuries may take place accidentally, this criterion must be used with caution.

We must add that persons found suspended have been previously killed by strangulation or other violence, and by poison.

DEATH BY STRANGULATION.

This mode of death is rare compared with death by hanging. It accounts for about 31 deaths a year, of which 16 are males and 15 females. Homicide by strangulation, though much more common than by hanging, is rare in adults, but common in children.

Strangulation differs from hanging only in the fact that the body is not suspended; but some cases of suicidal hanging in which the body touches the ground would be rightly set down to strangulation.

Strangling is usually effected by the uniform pressure of a ligature round the neck; but occasionally some hard substance is introduced into the folds of the ligature, and placed over the windpipe.

The mark on the neck will differ accordingly in the two cases,

* A great many cases, in which the bodies of suicides were found placed in every possible attitude, are given, illustrated by engravings, in an interesting paper in the fifth volume of the "Annales d'Hygiène."

being oblique and high up in death by hanging, circular and low down in death by strangulation. From this rule, however, we must except those cases of hanging in which the cord is firmly fixed, and those in which the body touches the ground; and those rare cases of strangulation in which it happens that the ligature is fixed somewhat obliquely. The mark in hanging, therefore, may happen to be circular, and that in strangulation more or less oblique. A foreign body in the folds of the ligature would be indicated by the greater size and distinctness of the bruise over the windpipe.

Another difference between the two modes of death is, that in strangulation much more force is used, rendering the mark on the neck more distinct, and the injury to the subjacent parts greater. This will be especially the case in homicidal strangulation, for the murderer generally uses unnecessary violence.

Frequently, also, there are wounds and bruises of other parts of the body indicative of struggling; and to the same cause are to be attributed certain appearances described by Tardieu as occurring in strangulation more frequently than in any other form of asphyxia. These are punctated ecchymoses on the conjunctiva, face, neck, and upper part of the chest; and interstitial emphysema due to rupture of some of the superficial air-cells of the lungs. Sometimes also apoplectic extravasations are found on the surface of the lungs of much larger extent than the capillary ecchymoses which occur more particularly in simple suffocation.

The same questions arise in respect of strangulation as of hanging—viz.:

Was death caused by strangulation?

Was the strangulation accidental, suicidal, or homicidal?

Was death caused by strangulation?—A cord applied a few hours after death would not produce so much bruise as would result from its application during life; and the turgescence of the face and characteristic post-mortem appearances would be wanting. It is only, therefore, in suicides, and in the scarcely conceivable case of slight force being used by the murderer, or death taking place suddenly, from shock or syncope, that the appearances produced by a cord applied during life could resemble those due to its application after death; and the same is true of direct pressure on the windpipe. As, moreover, hanging is known to be a common suicidal act, the murderer is not likely to simulate strangulation in order to hide the real mode of death. It is much more likely that, having strangled his victim, he would attempt concealment by suspending the body or placing it in a position suggestive of suicide.

In the well-known case of Bartholomew Pourpre, the deceased was first strangled and then suspended, and the mark of the cord was found at the lower part of the neck, while the teeth knocked in, and the bloody mouth, showed the violence that had been used.

The murderers of Sir Edmondbury Godfrey, after strangling him near Somerset House with a twisted handkerchief very forcibly applied, hid the body for a time, and then carried it to Islington, threw it into a ditch, passed his own sword through him, and laid his gloves and other articles of dress on the bank, so as to create a belief that he had committed suicide. The absence of blood from the wound, though the sword had passed through the heart, excited suspicion, which was fully confirmed by the discovery of a bruise, an inch broad, extending round the neck, and a fracture of the cervical vertebræ, which rendered the neck so flexible that it could be turned from one shoulder to the other. The face, which during life was remarkably pale, was livid and suffused, and the eyes bloodshot.

In 1892, a medical man, Mr. Kenvain, was throttled in Southwark by three men, one of whom placed his left hand over the mouth of his victim, and with his right compressed the throat. Shortly after the attack Kenvain was discovered, but he died almost immediately. The post-mortem examination showed only a slight crescentic mark on the neck, with its convexity downwards, a little to the right and below the cricoid cartilage. The scalp showed many ecchymoses, and the features were leaden and livid; blood was extravasated along the larynx and trachea, the hyoid bone, the thyroid and cricoid cartilages were fractured, the lungs were emphysematous, the air-cells contained blood, the heart had both its ventricles nearly empty, and the auricles were not distended. (*Guy's Hosp. Reports*, 1892.)

Was the strangulation accidental, suicidal, or homicidal?—That strangulation, like hanging, may be **accidental**, is proved by the following cases :—

An ingenious young man having nearly lost the use of his arms, used to move a heavy weight by a cord passed round his neck.

One morning, soon after he went to his room, his sister found him sitting in a chair quite dead, with the cord twisted round the neck. The deceased must have tried to move the weight in the usual way, but it had slipped behind, and so strangled him. (Smith.)

In July, 1839, Elizabeth Kenchan, an extremely dissipated, drunken, and disorderly woman, went to bed intoxicated, with her bonnet on, and in the morning was found strangled in its strings. She had fallen out of bed, her bonnet became fixed between the bedstead and the wall, and she, being too drunk to loosen the strings, was strangled.

In a few cases, then, death by strangulation has been accidental; but if death did not take place in this way, the question is narrowed to the alternative of

Suicide or homicide.—Strangulation appears to be a suicidal act in about half the recorded cases. As it is hard for a man to strangle himself by the pressure of his own hands, even if aided by a ligature, he resorts to twisting. In one case (Orfila) two cravats were twisted several times round the neck; in another (Dunlop) a Malay used a small stick for the purpose; in a third case the handle of a pot was used. In the year 1838 a Mr. Watson, aged 88, strangled himself by placing a poker through the tie of his neckerchief and turning it round and round.

Strangulation by pressure of the hand on the trachea (throttling) may be safely assumed to be homicidal. A robust man seized another by the cravat, and pressed him firmly against a wall till he was dead. The face was found livid and swollen, and the features distorted; and there was considerable discoloration and depression at the seat of pressure. There were witnesses to the act, and the man was proved to be insane.

An unsuccessful attempt to attribute death to accidental throttling was made in 1763, in the case of Beddingfield. He was found dead in his bedroom, lying on his face on the floor, with one hand round his neck, and his wife and man-servant were charged with the murder. The medical testimony was very unsatisfactory, as no dissection had taken place, but it was proved that there were marks on the neck resembling those of fingers, One surgeon said there were marks of a thumb and *three* fingers; the other of a thumb and *four fingers;* while another witness saw only *two*, "which looked as if the blood was set in the skin."

One of the criminals after condemnation confessed that he had seized Beddingfield's throat with his left hand as he lay asleep, and that, though he struggled violently and made some noise, he soon accomplished his purpose.

The appearances caused by throttling, when great resistance is offered, may be inferred from the evidence of Mr. W. Wilson in the case of Hector M'Donald, convicted of the murder of his wife at Inveraray, April 1857. There was an abrasion on each side of the windpipe, five abrasions on the left, and three on the right arm; and the skin on the front and sides of the neck and on the upper part of the chest was blackened. On the throat were the marks of a thumb and three fingers. It was inferred that the throat had been grasped by the left hand, of which the wrist was pressed upon the chest, and that the right hand had grasped the left arm of the victim. The internal appearances were highly characteristic of death by asphyxia. The substance and membranes of the brain were injected; the lungs and right side of the heart contained a quantity of dark fluid blood; the left was nearly empty. All the internal viscera were healthy.

The following is a case of homicidal strangulation by a foreign body introduced into the ligature :—Dr. Clench, a London physician, was called out of bed by two men on the night of the 4th of January 1692, to visit a sick friend. He entered a hackney coach with them, and was driven about several streets in the city for an hour and a quarter. The men then left the coach and sent the driver on an errand. When he returned he found Dr. Clench sitting on the bottom of the coach, with his head on the cushion of the front seat. Thinking him in liquor, he shook him, but obtained no answer. He then called the watch, and they found him strangled by a coal wrapped in a handkerchief, and applied directly over the windpipe. The coachman had heard no noise while driving the carriage.

In the Dundee murder case, cunning and stupidity are well illustrated. (*Lancet,* 1889, vol. i. p. 696.) The prisoner went to the police station and stated that his wife had hung herself some days previously, but on inspection by the officer, no nail was found or any mark of one to which a rope could have been attached. The case was clearly one of homicidal strangulation, and the prisoner was convicted.

DEATH BY SUFFOCATION.

Under this head are comprised all cases of asphyxia not produced by direct pressure on the windpipe, with the exception of drowning, which has already been treated separately.

In the year 1892, 2195 deaths by suffocation occurred, of which 1197 were in males, and 998 in females. In this number are comprised a large number of infants (1654) killed by overlying or suffocated by bed-clothes, and others suffocated by their food or by gases, chiefly charcoal vapours.

Suffocation may take place in many ways.

The mouth and nostrils may be stopped accidentally or by force. A person in a state of helplessness, from whatever cause, may fall on the face, and be suffocated by water or loose earth; and new-born children by the discharges, by the bed-clothes, or by being overlaid. Suffocation by such forms of pressure is also a homicidal act.

Mechanical pressure on the chest.—This may be accidental, through the fall of earth or rubbish; or homicidal, the murderer pressing with his whole weight on the body, and at the same time compressing the windpipe with the hand, or pressing on the chest and closing the mouth and nostrils. Suffocation by pressure on the chest constituted part of the *peine forte et dure* of our ancient law. A risk of accidental suffocation by compression of the chest has been incurred in taking casts with plaster of Paris.

On the 14th of June 1837 twenty-three persons lost their lives in a crowd in the Champs de Mars, some deaths being due to suffocation, others to severe injury to the chest.

Closure of the glottis.—This also may be accidental, as in suffocation by food. When this happens in adults they are usually intoxicated, or in a fit. Thus Paris and Fonblanque quote the case of a patient who died in an epileptic fit after a heavy meal of pork, and the trachea contained a quantity of matter resembling the pork on which he had recently dined. This form of suffocation is not an uncommon termination of the general paralysis of the insane.

Accidental suffocation by small objects finding their way into the windpipe is not uncommon. The death of Anacreon, attributed to a grape-seed; that of Gilbert the poet to a piece of mutton; a case in which a piece of potato peel was found impacted in the rima glottidis, are cases in point. Of suffocation by irritating substances we have examples in a case of swallowing a bee in some honey; and another from slaked lime getting into the larynx. Small morbid growths, and the products of inflammation, have often sufficed to close this narrow passage.

Suffocation has also been often threatened and sometimes brought about by bodies impacted in the upper part of the gullet. Slaves, both in ancient and modern times, are alleged to have swallowed their tongues. Some articles of dress, such as a handkerchief, have been swallowed; and one determined suicide caused a fatal hæmorrhage by swallowing a cork bristling with sharp pins. The preparation is in the museum of King's College.

Suicidal suffocation by the vapours of charcoal are not common in England, but very frequent in France.

Suffocation is not often a homicidal act, at least in young and vigorous adults, for the force required is such as to reveal the cause of death by external marks and internal appearances; but when the body is very weak from any cause, as in the new-born infant, the old man, or the intoxicated, suffocation is not difficult to effect, and if not attended by great violence, might not betray itself by external or internal marks.

The post-mortem appearances present in well-marked death by suffocation are those of asphyxia. In the twenty-three persons suffocated in the crowd in the Champs de Mars, M. Ollivier found without exception the skin of the face and neck of a uniform violet tint, spotted with blackish ecchymoses. In nine, the eyes were bloodshot; in four, a bloody froth ran from the mouth and nostrils; in four, blood flowed from the nostrils, in three, from the ears; seven had fractures of the ribs; and two (females) fracture of the sternum. In sixteen bodies that were opened the blood was black and fluid, and filled all the large veins at the right side of the heart. The pulmonary tissue was mostly reddish-brown, and in three-quarters of each lung, posteriorly, there was a considerable accumulation of black and liquid blood; but there was no ecchymosis, either on the surface or in the substance of the lungs, except in one case. In all the cases in which the eyes were bloodshot, and in those in which blood flowed from the ears, the vessels of the pia mater and substance of the brain were gorged.

State of the Lungs.—In death by suffocation, especially in infants, the lungs are frequently congested; in other cases they are pale or congested only posteriorly. Emphysema and puncti-form ecchymoses are common appearances.

In most cases the surface of the lungs, instead of being smooth, is uneven or tuberculated, from partial vesicular or interstitial emphysema. A section into one of these patches shows that the parenchyma of the lung is affected.

The punctiform ecchymoses (Tardieu's spots) are found most commonly in children who have died of suffocation, but they may also occur in adults. They are minute spots on the pleura (visceral and costal), not confined to the surface of the lungs, for they may be observed on the thymus, the aorta, the heart, or the diaphragm; also on the surface of the abdominal viscera, and on the inner surface of the scalp. The surface of the lung looks as if it had been sprinkled with minute drops of a dark purple fluid. They are due to the rupture of the over-distended capillaries, and occur, according to Lükomsky, when the general blood-pressure is greatly increased by continued efforts to expire. Tardieu thought that they were diagnostic of death by suffocation as distinguished from other modes of death by asphyxia; but this opinion lacks confirmation, for they occur whenever a similar relation between the respiratory movements and the blood-pressure exists, and have been found in hanging, drowning, and suffocation, and in death from cerebral injuries. It seems, however, to be generally admitted that they occur most commonly in children killed by suffocation; and Ogston* is of opinion that their occurrence on the thymus, in clusters rather than singly, is strongly in favour of death by suffocation. They occur in the fœtus, from interruption of the placental circulation; and they are common in the lungs of new-born infants (see Fig. 26, p. 121). They indicate death from asphyxia, but not the way in which it was brought about.

The slight injuries caused by the suffocation of helpless people led to the selection of this mode of death by the persons engaged in the supply of bodies to the anatomical schools prior to the passing of the Anatomy Act. Burke, with his female accomplice,

* "Lectures on Med. Jurisp.," p. 554.

Macdougall, was tried at Edinburgh in 1828, and Bishop, with Williams and May, in London, in 1831.

Burke killed Margery Campbell by sitting on her body, covering the mouth and nostrils with one hand, and applying the other forcibly under the chin.

Fifty-nine hours after death, the eyes were closed; the features composed, as in deep sleep, red and somewhat swollen; the lips of a dark colour; and the eyes bloodshot. There was a little fluid blood on the left cheek, apparently from the nostrils; the tongue was not protruded or torn, but there was a slight laceration on the inside of the upper lip opposite the left eye-tooth; the cuticle under the chin was much ruffled, and the surface of the true skin, when laid bare, was dry and brown; but there was no bruise. The integuments, except on the face, were perfectly free from lividity. The joints were flaccid. There was no effusion of blood or laceration of the parts round the windpipe, and no injury of the cartilages, but the os hyoides and thyroid cartilage were further apart than usual. The following were the internal appearances: The membrane of the windpipe healthy, with here and there some tough mucus, not frothy, and a few bloody points between it and the membrane. The thoracic organs perfectly natural; the lungs remarkably so. The blood throughout the body black and fluid, and accumulated in the large veins, and in the right cavities of the heart. The abdominal viscera, with the exception of incipient disease of the liver, healthy. The brain also was quite healthy, and somewhat more turgescent than usual; and there were three extravasations of blood in the scalp, but without corresponding external bruise. There were some marks of violence on the limbs, considerable effusions of blood among the muscles of the neck, back, and loins, and on the sheath of the spinal cord. The posterior ligaments connecting the third and fourth cervical vertebræ were torn. A "handful" of clotted blood was found near the body.

In Carlo Ferrari, the victim of Bishop, the appearances from which suffocation might have been inferred were even less strongly marked. The face, it is true, was swollen and congested; the eyes bloodshot, and the lips tumid; but the lungs were quite healthy and not congested, the heart contracted, and all its cavities quite empty. But these exceptional appearances were explained by the fact that the murderers, after stupefying their victim with liquor lowered his body into a well, head downwards, keeping the mouth below the water. In this case, too, there were some extravasated blood under the scalp, among the muscles of the neck, and on the spinal cord. The fresh state of the body, the appearance of the countenance, and a wound on the left temple, combined to excite suspicion, and led to the committal and conviction of the murderers.

In both these cases death was certainly caused by suffocation, and yet the appearance of the bodies was not such as to lead at once to the conclusion that death had happened in this way. The medical examiners in both cases were inclined to ascribe the deaths to the injury done to the spine, which was afterwards proved to have been occasioned after death by the forcible doubling up of the bodies in packing them.

In allusion to the opinion that the signs of suffocation are so strongly marked as of themselves to arrest attention, Christison, speaking of the woman Campbell, says that "no person of skill, who had been told that murder was probable, but the manner of death unknown, could have failed to remark signs that would raise a suspicion of suffocation. But if he had not known that suspicions were entertained, he might have inspected the body even minutely, and yet neglected the signs in question. Every one conversant with pathological anatomy must be familiar with similar appearances as arising from various natural diseases ; and they were present in the body of a man who died of dysentery, the 'vascularity of the conjunctivæ and the contusions on the legs' being 'the only difference.' "*

* Cases and Observations in Medical Jurisprudence : *Ed. Med. and Surg. Journal*, vol. xxxi. p. 243, 1829.

CHAPTER III.

WOUNDS AND MECHANICAL INJURIES.

THIS chapter treats all injuries inflicted by mechanical means, except the several forms of death by suffocation examined in the previous chapter, and injuries by fire and by lightning, reserved for separate examination in Chapter VI.

All injuries, therefore, which one man inflicts on another, whether by cutting or bruising instruments, by his own person, or by forcing him against an obstacle, will have to be considered under this head. For the punishment of all such injuries when maliciously inflicted, the statute law makes provision, no less than for stabbing, cutting, shooting, drowning, strangling, and suffocating, by the insertion of the words "or shall by any means whatsoever wound or cause any grievous bodily harm to any person" and "by any means other than those specified," &c., and "with or without any weapon or instrument," &c. (§§ 11, 15, and 20 of 24 and 25 Vict. cap. c.), and further the case of Reg. v. Frill (July 31, 1890, Liverpool, Mr. Justice Williams) is interesting as showing the far-reaching character of the law in these cases. This was the case of a woman, Mary Frill, who had been convicted under the Summary Jurisdiction Act for an assault upon Carr. This person subsequently died as the result of the injuries; a plea of "autrefois convict" was made, setting out the fact of the prisoner's conviction for assault, and alleging that the acts constituting the alleged felonious killing were the acts which constituted the assault. The plea was not allowed.

In examining this large subject the following arrangement will be adopted. The several kinds of mechanical injury will be separately considered; then the questions common to all such injuries; then the way in which they affect the more important organs of the body.

Three kinds of mechanical injury will have to be examined in turn; wounds as commonly understood, gunshot wounds, and mechanical injuries not usually designated as "wounds."

The old surgical definition of a wound* makes it to consist in a solution of continuity. Mechanical injuries, therefore, may be conveniently divided into such as are without solution of continuity and such as are with solution of continuity. The first includes *contusions, concussions, simple fractures, dislocations*, and *sprains*. The second comprises *incisions, punctures*, and *lacerations, compound fractures*, and *gun-shot wounds*.

Each class of injuries, whatever the parts affected, has some points common to all the forms of violence included in the class. Thus, almost all injuries affecting the deeper-seated parts are accompanied by external traces of the force that produced them, whether it caused a solution of continuity or not. So that in most cases we shall have traces of the injury on the *surface*, and it will therefore be necessary to examine minutely the subject of bruises and incisions involving the external parts of the body.

The subject will be best examined under the following heads :—

I. CONTUSED WOUNDS AND INJURIES UNACCOM-PANIED BY SOLUTION OF CONTINUITY.

II. INCISED WOUNDS AND WOUNDS ACCOMPANIED BY A SOLUTION OF CONTINUITY.

III. GUNSHOT WOUNDS.

IV. QUESTIONS COMMON TO ALL FORMS OF ME-CHANICAL INJURY.

V. WOUNDS AS THEY AFFECT DIFFERENT PARTS OF THE BODY.

VI. THE DETECTION OF BLOOD-STAINS, HAIR, ETC.

I. CONTUSED WOUNDS, AND INJURIES UNACCOM-PANIED BY SOLUTION OF CONTINUITY.

A blow with a blunt instrument causes an appearance on the surface commonly known as a bruise, in scientific language an ecchymosis. It consists in a discoloration of the skin produced

---

* "A wound is a solution of continuity in any part of the body suddenly made by anything that cuts or tears, with a division of the skin." "By the word skin I understand not only the external cutis, but also the inward membranes of the gullet, ventricle, guts, bladder, urethra, and womb, all of which are capable of wounds from sharp instruments, either swallowed or thrust into them."— WISEMAN's "Chirugical Treatises," book v. chap. I.

by extravasation of blood into the cellular tissue. When this happens in the superficial parts, and especially in the lax and yielding skin, the colour shows itself at once; but when deeper-seated, days may elapse before the skin becomes discoloured, and then it is not blue, as in superficial parts, but of a violet, greenish, or yellowish hue: nor is it always immediately over the seat of injury, the point where the extravasation becomes visible being conditioned by the arrangement of the fascia and cellular tissue offering resistance in some directions but not in others.

The blue colour is not fully developed at once, but continues to deepen for five or six hours. When blood ceases to flow from the broken vessels, serum is effused, and inflammation is set up, and thus the bruise is enlarged. Its colour also undergoes a change, passing from deep blue to shades of green, yellow, and lemon colour, such colour-changes being consequent upon chemical changes in the hæmoglobin of the blood. After a further interval the effused fluids are absorbed, and the colours first fade and then wholly disappear. If the injury has been severe, the inflammation runs on to suppuration, forming an abscess if deep, an ulcer if superficial.

The change of colour begins at the circumference, where the effused fluids are scanty, and travels inwards towards the centre, where they are abundant, and where the deep blue colour often remains after the rest of the bruise has completely changed its appearance. In bruises of any extent, and in parts that contain much blood, coagula are formed.

The extent of the bruise and the rapidity of its changes will depend on the force used, the size and character of the weapon, the age, constitution, and health of the sufferer, the full or empty state of the vessels, and the tension or laxity of the skin. A boxer in training would scarcely be marked by a blow that would disfigure a person in ordinary health; and in severe cases of scurvy the lightest touch causes a bruise closely resembling that produced in healthy persons by greater violence.

As the form of a bruise is in part determined by the shape of the weapon, it often furnishes strong presumptive evidence. The subjects of death by hanging, strangulation, and suffocation have furnished good examples of this correspondence of bruises with their cause, and in one case (Starkie, "Law of Evidence") a blow on the face given in self-defence with the key of the house door, caused a bruise which corresponded in shape to the wards of the key, and served to identify the man who had committed the assault.

The discolorations of a bruise are not confined to the cellular tissue, but involve the substance of the true skin. Bruises are thus distinguished from cadaveric lividity. (See p. 291.)

But even severe blows do not produce marks of injury on the surface when the parts beneath are soft and yielding. Thus blows on the abdomen which rupture the viscera do not always bruise the skin, though they sometimes cause the effusion of blood between the muscles. On the other hand, when severe injuries of hard parts, such as fractures of bone, are unattended by a bruise, there is a strong presumption against their having been caused by a blow.

Can the appearance of a bruise be produced after death ?

This question is answered by Christison's experiments, from which it appears that, up to two hours after death, and in rare cases three hours and a quarter, appearances may be produced more or less resembling bruises inflicted during life; blood is effused into the cellular tissue on the surface of the cutis, and even into its substance; and the blood coagulates.

Distinction between bruises inflicted during life and after death.—In certain cases this distinction is easy. If there is much swelling, any change of colour, or any sign of inflammation, the bruise must have been inflicted during life.

If on incising the bruise the effusion is found to be considerable and the clots large, there is a strong presumption that it was inflicted during life. So also if the cutis is discoloured by blood effused into its texture. This is a valuable diagnostic mark, except in the case of bruises inflicted a few minutes after death, when, judging from the analogy of incised wounds, we may expect the same appearances.

As the same effusion of blood which on the surface constitutes a bruise, may when it occurs in deeper-seated parts, leave little or no trace upon the skin, it is important to ascertain whether such deeper effusions may take place after death as well as during life. This question has been answered in the affirmative. In the body of Margery Campbell, the victim of Burke (see p. 345), there were marks of severe injury to the back, to which Christison was at first inclined to attribute her death; and semi-fluid blood was found under the trapezius muscle, near the inferior angle of the scapula, and in the cervical, dorsal, and left lumbar regions; but there was no corresponding bruise on the skin. The posterior ligaments of the vertebræ were ruptured, but there was no fracture. On the sheath of the spinal cord, opposite the rupture, there was a mass of semi-fluid black blood an inch wide, and about the thickness of a penny, and from this a thin layer of blood extended along the posterior surface of the sheath as far as the lowest dorsal vertebra. The spinal cord was not injured, nor was there any blood under its sheath. Christison proved that all these marks of violence might be produced seventeen hours after death, by bending the head forcibly on the chest. In the body of Carlo Ferrari, also, five or six ounces of coagulated blood were found among the deep-seated muscles of the neck, from the occiput to the last cervical vertebra; and there was a large quantity of fluid blood in the upper and lower part of the spinal canal, exterior to the sheath of the cord, but no blood within the sheath; nor had the vertebræ, or their ligaments, or the cord itself, suffered any injury. The confession of the criminals showed that these injuries to the spine were produced after death.

The difficulty of determining whether a bruise was inflicted during life or soon after death is much increased if putrefaction has set in; for it exaggerates the appearance of injury, and produces great alterations of consistence and colour; while the pressure of the gases evolved may cause copious outpourings of blood through ruptured vessels. This was well shown in the body of a man who had died of apoplexy. The veins of both arms had been opened, but no more blood had flowed during life. After death, however, an abundant hæmorrhage took place from the wounded vessels (G.).

In a case which occurred at Paris (p. 51), the effusion of blood caused by strangling was discovered as a black mass twenty years after death. But the cord was round the neck, and removed the difficulty which might otherwise have existed.

The same observations apply to fractures, and in nearly the same degree. A fracture produced soon after death, and one produced just before life is extinct, would probably present very nearly the same appearances; while a fracture caused some time before death would be readily distinguished by the inflammation set up about it.

Fractures may be detected long after death; in the body of Clarke, the victim of Eugene Aram, the indented fracture of the temporal bone after the lapse of thirteen years.

II. INCISED WOUNDS, AND WOUNDS ACCOMPANIED BY A SOLUTION OF CONTINUITY.

Under this head are comprised incised, punctured, and lacerated wounds; gunshot wounds being treated separately.

The immediate obvious consequences of wounds with solution of continuity are hæmorrhage and retraction of their edges; the remote effects those of inflammation and its sequelæ. In a recent incised wound, inflicted during life, there is copious hæmorrhage, the cellular tissue is filled with blood, there are coagula between the lips of the wound, and the edges are everted. After from eighteen to twenty-four hours there are the signs of inflammation —increased redness, swelling, and effusion of coagulable lymph.

As a rule, incised wounds, whether caused by cutting or slashing, are fusiform in shape, owing to the retraction of the tissues in the middle, and especially so when muscular fibres have been divided transversely. Incised wounds usually commence abruptly and terminate gradually or tail off; sometimes, especially in cut-throat, the wound ends in two or more points, thus indicating the direction in which the instrument was drawn.

Incised wounds do not correspond in shape to the weapon which inflicted them, the wound being broader than the cutting edge.

A close resemblance to an incised wound may be caused by a blunt instrument or by a fall, in firm resisting parts; as, for instance, on the integument covering the skull.

Copious hæmorrhage affords a strong presumption in favour of a wound having been inflicted during life, especially if the body is fresh. Scanty hæmorrhage, or the entire absence of it, as in the case of Sir Edmondbury Godfrey (p. 339), supplies an equally strong reason for attributing death to some other cause. But lacerated and severe gun-shot wounds form an exception to this rule. In the case recorded by Cheselden, of a man's arm torn off by a windmill, and in one reported by Mr. Bransby Cooper, there was scarcely any hæmorrhage. On the other hand, very considerable hæmorrhage may take place after death, and especially when putrefaction is set up, if any large vein happens to be wounded.

In the case of incised as of contused wounds, it is important to determine whether the appearances found in wounds inflicted during life may be produced after death.

Characters of wounds produced after death.—The experiments of Orfila on the dog have shown that the appearances proper to incised wounds inflicted during life may be produced immediately after death; and the experiments of Dr. Taylor, made on limbs recently amputated, show to what degree the resemblance may be carried.

When the incision was made two minutes after the removal, there was immediate considerable retraction of the skin, protrusion of the adipose substance, and scanty flow of blood; and after twenty-four hours the edges were found red, bloody, and everted; the skin somewhat flaccid; a small quantity of blood escaped on separating the edges; no coagula adhered to the muscles; but at the bottom of the wound were several loose coagula.

After an interval of ten minutes a second experiment was performed. The edges of the wound were slightly everted; scarcely any blood escaped; and twenty-four hours afterwards the edges were pale and perfectly collapsed, and at the bottom of the wound were found a few coagula.

When the wound was not made till two or three hours had elapsed, a small quantity of liquid blood was effused, and no clots were found. The edges of an incised wound made twenty-four hours after death were yielding, inelastic, in close approximation, and free from coagula.

Lacerated wounds combine the characters of incised and contused wounds, being attended with less hæmorrhage than the former, and less discoloration than the latter. The edges are generally torn, but, as above stated, though caused by blunt instruments or falls, they may be sharp and defined. They seldom correspond in shape with the cause. The distinction between such wounds inflicted during life and after death is less easily made.

Punctured wounds are intermediate between incised and lacerated wounds, resembling the former when inflicted with a sharp instrument, and being often accompanied by profuse hæmorrhage; but when made with a blunt object, being more like lacerated wounds, and causing little loss of blood. The form depends on the shape of the weapon and the direction of the blow. They are generally smaller than the weapon. They resemble incised wounds if the weapon is a broad, two-edged blade. Wounds, when made by a perpendicular stroke, correspond to the breadth of the weapon, but a blow struck obliquely produces a longer wound. Weapons with a thick back and sharp edge cause wounds of a corresponding shape. Triangular weapons, such as bayonets, cause triangular wounds.

It must be remembered, however, that the same weapon may produced differently shaped wounds on different parts, according to the tissue penetrated and the amount of retraction which ensues.

Sword wounds traversing the body have a large depressed orifice of entrance, and a small raised orifice of exit; but this condition may be reversed when the weapon is drawn out, especially if it is rough from rust or otherwise.

The chief danger of punctured wounds is from injury to internal organs or penetration of internal closed cavities, such as the pleura.

III. GUN-SHOT WOUNDS.

When a bullet passes through the atmosphere, it drives before it a wave of compressed air; this, however, has no real bursting effect, inasmuch as it exerts but very feeble pressure, and is easily reflected from surfaces of but moderate density. A bullet discharged from a rifle has a certain spin communicated to it, consequent upon the rifling of the barrel. This is generally thought to cause a considerable amount of disturbance in the interior of moist substances, and by a series of experiments by Mr. Victor Horsley it has been shown that the rotation of the bullet persists to the end, when it has taken its course through the air and then entered a soft substance, and, further, the twist is proportionally more pronounced as the forward movement is lost; the rotatory movement is also maintained even when the projectile is completely deformed, but so far as distinctive effects on the brain are concerned, but little is to be ascribed to rotation.

As the result of a bullet wound, there are two sets of factors to be considered: (*a*) Those due to the bullet; (1) its momentum, (2) its sectional area, and (3) the heat developed; and (*b*) those due to the physical constitution of the penetrated solid.

(*a*) Factors due to the bullet:

(1) Momentum.—As regards this, the particles of any substance in

front of the bullet are hurried forward, and as thus the size of the moving mass is increased, such particles practically constituting a larger projectile, as a consequence much destruction follows. This is well illustrated by Delorme in the case of firing a bullet into a book, the laceration of the pages being successively increased, although the momentum of the bullet is steadily diminishing. This point is obviously of great importance in bullet wounds of the head when discs of bone are forced through the brain.

(2) Sectional area.—The crushing effect of a bullet will be proportional to its diameter, and seeing that a bullet on striking an iron plate, by its compression gives rise to a hole much greater than its diameter, on leaving the rifle, it becomes a question for consideration what proportion of the damage done is due to deformation of the projectile on its striking the body.

(3) As regards the heat developed.—This is probably greatly exaggerated and calls for no comment.

(b) Factors due to the physical constitution of the solid penetrated.

Huguier, suggested, as the result of his experiments on lung, liver, &c., that the lateral disturbance was occasioned by the presence in the tissues of large quantities of water, and that the energy of the projectile being imparted to the particles of water, caused their dispersion in a hydrodynamic manner; and Kocher, in 1874-76, proved that the effect was really a hydrodynamic one; one of his most striking experiments being, to take two tin canisters of equal size and strength, the one being filled with dry lint, the other with lint saturated with water. On firing a bullet of moderate velocity through these canisters, the one containing the dry lint was simply perforated, the other burst explosively. And further, Kocher showed that if a bullet was fired into a skull containing water, not only would the sutures burst, but this bursting would be greatest on the side of the entry of the bullet. From these facts we are led to conclude that, when a bullet strikes the skull transversely, it first causes a depression of the bone over an area greater than the diameter of the uninjured bullet; secondly, as a result of this cause slight tension of the fluid contents of the skull; and thirdly, on the entrance of the bullet into the skull, general displacement of the contents follows, a severe rise of pressure occurs, most marked on the side of entry of the bullet, and this tends to burst the skull, or, if not, to be reflected on the brain, this being compressed wherever an unyielding surface is found.

Applying these principles, and by several ingenious experiments, Mr. Horsley has shown that the fatal phenomena of a gun-shot wound of the cerebral hemisphere is at first, and above all, arrest of respiration, and when it is remembered that the medulla oblongata contains the chief respiratory centre, as well as the origin of the pneumogastric nerve, which has the power of slowing the heart, and that this is subjected to pressure when a bullet traverses transversely the brain, the arrest of respiration, with the slowing and ultimate failure of the heart's action, is explained. Further, the pressure on the medulla oblongata is increased subsequently by the wounding of the blood-vessels, and consequent extravasation.

Gun-shot wounds may be defined as contused or lacerated wounds; contused when the projectile does not penetrate, lacerated when it enters or traverses the body. When penetrating they are accompanied by loss of substance, and partake of the character of deep punctured wounds. Their gravity is proportionate to the region of the body struck or traversed, to the structures injured, and to the size, form, nature, density, and velocity of the projectile, as well as to the serious consequences of inflammation they induce, and to the introduction of foreign bodies—e.g., the projectile itself and portions of clothing.

A distinction must be drawn between wounds caused by bullets and those by small shot.

The modern rifle bullet is conical, either at the apex alone, or ovoid, as in the needle-gun ; it differs from the old round bullet in its greater initial velocity and penetrating power; the resulting wound being therefore more serious. A bullet may strike the body tangentially, causing a contusion, grooving the skin and subcutaneous tissue, or passing beneath the skin for a greater or less distance, causing the so-called seton-wound. In the majority of cases it traverses a portion of the body—a limb, or a part of the trunk. In its course it may wound only the soft parts or the great vessels, causing hæmorrhage; it may injure nerves, or greatly comminute and fissure bones. If a bone be struck by a bullet at full speed, a round opening, with well-defined margins, is punched in it, while spreading from the opening are fissures; in other cases, with less velocity, the bone may be partially fractured, indented, fissured, or simply contused.

In the soft parts the entrance wound is sharply defined and smaller in area than the bullet, the edges being contused, inverted, and depressed. The exit wound is irregular, with everted margins, like an ordinary lacerated wound. If the velocity be less, the wounds are less regular and larger. A similar difference between entrance and exit may be seen in the clothes.

The bullet, shot, or wadding discharged from fire-arms at short distances sometimes lodges in the body, sometimes traverses it. When it lodges it often furnishes conclusive evidence. The bullet may have been cast in a mould, or the wadding formed by printed paper or other material, in the possession of the person who fired the shot. It may even happen that the composition of the bullet, or the mode of making it, is peculiar. In medico-legal cases, therefore, the contents of a gun-shot wound should be carefully examined and preserved.

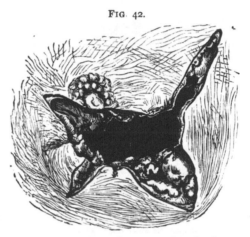

FIG. 42.

Pistol-shot (suicide). Large star-shaped entrance wound. Two-thirds natural size. (Hofmann).

A gun-shot track is not a cylinder, the opening in the skin being smaller in area than that of the bullet; in the aponeurosis there is often a mere slit. Bullets which lodge in the body are often turned out of their direct course by contact with a bone, with a contracting muscle, a tense fascia, or a tendon. Thus (to give examples from the practice of Richard Wiseman), a bullet entered the cheek, and was cut out from the back of the neck; a second entered the outside of the small of the leg, and was found on the inside of the thigh above the knee; and a third entered the outside of the arm, and was cut out below the scapula. In some cases the bullet has struck the head or abdomen, and after traversing the half-circumference of the part, has been found lodged, or to have passed out, at the opposite point. Again, bullets may be split into two or more fragments by striking a bone, and these fragments may either traverse the body or lodge in it. If they lodge, they may be found to have taken the same eccentric course as the undivided bullet in the cases just cited: if they traverse, they may occasion more than one wound of exit resembling that caused by a single bullet.

When a bullet takes a direct course through the body (that is to say, when it is not deflected), the character of the two apertures, coupled with the direction of the line which joins them, may serve to indicate the posture of the body when the wound was received.

FIG. 43.

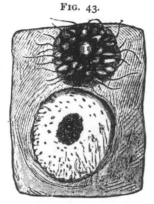

FIG. 44.

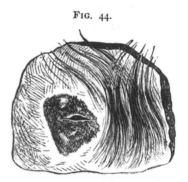

Entrance wound of a chamber-revolver, under left nipple. Suicide. Natural size. The wound is surrouuded by a large zone flecked with pow-der grains. (Hofmann.)

Wound by revolver bullet, simulating a cut by a sharp instrument. Natural size. (Hofmann.)

So also when, after traversing a wooden paling, or a window, it strikes a wall beyond, the line of flight and spot from which the shot was fired may be determined.

A revolver-bullet fired close to the body may produce an exten-sively lacerated wound (as in Fig. 42), or a round aperture with a surrounding contusion (Fig. 43), or a slit like the wound of a knife, but with a surrounding ecchymosis (as in Fig. 44). The skin and clothing may be blackened or burnt.

Small shot discharged close to the body, and striking it at right angles, may cause a round clean wound not easily distinguished from one produced by a bullet; but at the distance of a foot or more the shot scatter, and the wound is irregular. At the distance of three feet the shot are so scattered that it is not possible to confound the injury with one caused by a bullet; the exit wound is very irregular, and is sievelike at the margin, owing to the separate exit of pellets of shot. In these wounds some of the shot lodge in the body, and when fired close, or within a short distance, there are marks of burning on the skin and clothing. Fire-arms loaded with wadding, and fired close to the body, or within a few inches, may produce severe and even fatal penetrating wounds, and even at the distance of a foot may give rise to extensive superficial injuries. The unconsumed powder, when fire-arms loaded only with powder are discharged close to the body, may produce the same injuries as small shot.

From what has been said above of the complicated nature of gun-shot wounds, it is obvious that they are very dangerous. They may prove fatal immediately, or soon, by injury to a vital organ, such as the brain or heart; by shock or hæmorrhage; and, after a long interval, by secondary hæmorrhage, by erysipelas, by tetanus, or by the inflammation and extensive suppuration or gangrene following the injury to the parts.

The same medico-legal questions (such as the more or less dangerous character of the wound, the effect of the treatment adopted, and of the subsequent conduct of the wounded person, on the issue of the injury, and the amount of locomotion possible after it) arise in gun-shot as in other wounds.

The question whether the wound was the result of **accident, suicide,** or **homicide,** may also be raised respecting these, in common with other wounds. As a general rule, accidental wounds, whether inflicted by the wounded person in loading or in the act of carrying a loaded piece, or by another person pointing at him a piece supposed not to be loaded, or walking or shooting in his company, have the characters of wounds caused by discharges near the person; but these they share with suicidal wounds. Suicidal wounds, however, have a character which accidental wounds often, and homicidal wounds sometimes lack, of being inflicted in front, on the head or region of the heart. To this rule, however, some suicidal gun-shot wounds form an exception, the weapon being directed to the back of the head. As a general rule, too, the suicide fires only one shot; but suicides have been known to fire two pistols, and even to resort to fire-arms after the failure of incised wounds. In some cases the suicide is found in a room secured from within, with the weapon still grasped in the hand, and when the priming was of powder, with the hand stained by it.

Some information may be gained as to the time when the shot

was fired, though the conclusions can only be regarded as approximate. If the interior of the barrel blackens the finger introduced into it, and is free from crystals of protosulphate of iron, or rust, and the solution has a yellowish colour, smells strongly of sulphuretted hydrogen, and gives a black precipitate with acetate of lead, the weapon has not been discharged more than *two hours*. If the colour of the interior is less dark, but contains neither rust nor crystals of ferrous sulphate, but the solution gives traces of sulphuric acid—tested with acetate of lead or chloride of barium—the time that has elapsed is more than two hours, but *less than twenty-four* hours. When numerous spots of rust are visible in the interior, and when the solution gives indications of iron—tested by ferricyanide of potassium—*at least twenty-four hours, possibly six days*, have elapsed. When the rust is more copious, and the solution no longer gives iron reactions, at *least ten days, possibly fifty days*, have elapsed since the discharge.

One of the most interesting cases of gun-shot wounds of recent years, is that known as the Ardlamont Case, the main features of which are as follows :—

On the 10th of August 1893, a Lieutenant Hamborough, staying at Ardlamont House, Tighnabruaich, Scotland, was out shooting with Messrs. Monson and Scott; during the morning, Monson returned home for assistance, stating that while the party were passing through a wood and separated from each other, he and Scott heard the report of a gun, and on coming up discovered Hamborough lying dead at the foot of a sunk fence. A medical man who was summoned found a large wound behind the right ear, and after an investigation by the Procurator Fiscal, the body was taken to Ventnor and there buried.

On August 28th, Monson was arrested, and in December tried at Edinburgh, for the murder of Hamborough, the alleged motive for the murder being that Monson was in pecuniary difficulties, and had a large interest in certain life insurances the deceased had been induced by him to effect.

In this, as in all cases of death from gun-shot wounds, in order to determine whether it was one of accident, suicide, or murder, it was important to know—(1) The position, direction, and character of the wound; (2) The position of the body; (3) The position of the weapon relative to the body.

Skilled evidence was only obtainable on the first of these points,

inasmuch as the body had been removed to the house before
medical assistance was summoned. The body was buried after a
preliminary inquiry, the death being assumed to be accidental.
Suspicion subsequently being aroused, the body was exhumed

FIG. 45.

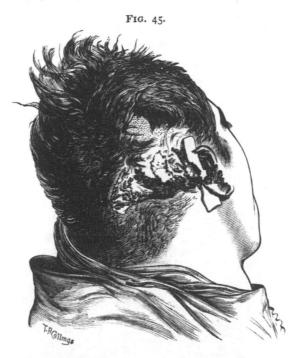

A view of the wound of the soft parts, a piece of paper is placed
under the ear. (From a photograph.)

twenty-five days after death, when the following were the chief
points noted :—

The features were somewhat swollen, but admitted of ready
identification, and the body generally was well preserved. The
wound was roughly triangular in shape (Fig. 45), the apex one inch
below and slightly anterior to the occipital protuberance, the base
towards the face on a level with the ear, of which the pinna was
wanting for 1½ inches in the centre of the edge ; the general direction of the wound was almost horizontal, the edges at the apex
bevelled and clean cut, but anteriorly they were more ragged ; in
front of the auditory meatus there was a small wound which communicated with the larger wound behind the ear. There were no
individual pellets beyond the edges of the wound. In the skull, near
the apex of the scalp wound, at a distance of 1½ inches from the

external auditory meatus, there was (Fig. 46) an irregular oval aperture, the posterior margin of which was slightly grooved as if from pellets, and bevelled at the expense of the inner table; the petrous portion of the temporal bone was ploughed, and extensive fissures with a general direction forwards from the original aperture crossed the right side, one passing across the base and involving the foramen magnum. The dura mater below the wound was extensively torn and the lateral sinus lacerated.

From these data, to which must be added the injury to the trees,

FIG. 46.

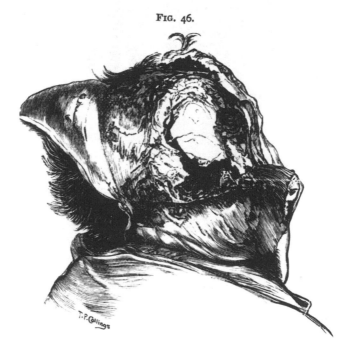

A view of the injuries to the skull, the soft parts having been reflected.
(From a photograph.)

the experts had to determine the direction from which the shot came, and the distance at which it had been fired.

With regard to the first point, both sides agreed that the injury was due to a glancing shot striking the skull obliquely from behind. As to distance, various experiments were made of the shooting of the particular guns used—two breech-loaders, a twenty-bore and a twelve-bore—and with the object of comparing the three powders, viz., Black, Schultze, and Amberite.

Trials of the guns were made at various distances, from one to twenty-four feet, in order to get what is technically known as a "pattern" of the gun, but the guns were somewhat worn and otherwise peculiar, and the results obtained could not be relied on in future cases.

Up to three feet the individual pellets did not show on the target (cardboard being found to be better than wood, which splintered), they became evident on, but not beyond, the edges of the central hole at three to four feet, while at nine feet there was a zone of pellets one inch from the edge of the central hole, the scattering increasing till at twelve to fifteen feet an open "pattern" was obtained.

With the different powders, the difference in "pattern" produced

FIG. 47.

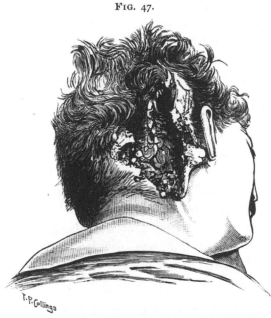

The result of an experiment with the 12-bore gun loaded with Amberite and fired at two feet distance.

was slight; it was demonstrated that singeing and scorching was not obtained with Amberite powder at any distance, a yellow discoloration occurred with nitro powders, and, in addition, a singeing with the black powder at distances nearer than three feet; and with Schultze, as with Black, there was engraining of the part with unburnt powder when nearer than three feet, the grains being, in the case of the Schultze, of light yellow colour.

The results of the experiments made both by the Crown and the defence experts practically coincided, although their opinions differed as to the distance to be inferred from them; the former deciding on nine feet as the probable distance, the latter holding that the shot might have been fired as close as a few inches, but certainly not farther than four feet from the head.

The prisoner stated that on coming up to the scene of the accident with Scott, they together lifted the body from the ditch where they found it lying, to the top of the sunk fence.

The Crown contended that the injuries observed to the trees in the immediate neighbourhood fixed the distance of the shot at nine feet, but for such injuries to the trees to have been inflicted at the time of the alleged murder it would have been necessary that the body had throughout laid on the top of the sunk fence instead of in the ditch, and while the Crown argued that the absence of blood and broken bracken in the ditch opposed the view that the body had laid there, the defence asserted that, as the grass was at the time wet, any blood flowing would have been washed into the ground. There was a further contention on the part of the Crown as to the possibility of Scott (who disappeared immediately after the accident) and Monson being able to lift the body the height of the wall without leaving traces of blood on their own hands or clothes, or on the clothes of the deceased. The medical witnesses for the Crown also considered that, though the hæmorrhage would have been oozing in character, it must have been profuse, and have set in immediately on account of the injury to the lateral sinus; while by the defence it was maintained that the wound in the sinus might have been temporarily plugged by a piece of bone which was displaced by the lifting. The prisoner was discharged on a verdict of "Not Proven."

IV. QUESTIONS COMMON TO ALL FORMS OF MECHANICAL INJURY.

There are three questions common to all forms of mechanical injury:—**Was it inflicted during life? Was it the cause of death?** and **Was it accidental, suicidal, or homicidal?** The first question has been already examined; the second and third remain to be discussed.

Was the wound the cause of death?—The answer to this question presents no difficulty when a man in the enjoyment of perfect health receives a severe injury, and dies before sufficient time has elapsed for disease to set in, or neglect or unskilful treatment to prove injurious. But when the interval is considerable between the receipt of the injury and the fatal event, such complications may arise, and make the answer to the question difficult.

But the abnormal formation or unusual situation of the part injured may entail a fatal result from an injury otherwise harmless. Of abnormal formation, the case of a boy caught robbing an orchard, whose death was caused by a blow intended as a simple chastisement, on a skull preternaturally thin, is a good illustration ; of abnormal situation, that of an inguinal hernia injured by a kick, or the fatal hæmorrhage caused by a blow on the loins over the seat of a kidney containing a jagged calculus; or a large abscess behind the ear ruptured by the same means.

To this class of cases also belong those sudden deaths which follow falls or blows too slight to account for the fatal result by the direct injury they occasion, death being really caused by the rupture of a vessel on the brain, or of an aneurism, in both of which cases it is possible to attribute death to the excitement of the struggle as well as to the fall or blow. Also, those cases of latent effusion on the brain or into the cavities of the chest which might prove suddenly fatal even in the absence of violence, but are very likely to cause death under the influence of shock.

In these cases the injury is inflicted in ignorance of the existence of any cause by which, though comparatively slight, it might be rendered mortal. To all other cases, such as those of young, feeble, or aged persons, and pregnant women, the English law, as laid down by Lord Hale, will apply : " It is sufficient to prove that the death of the party was *accelerated* by the malicious act of the prisoner, although the former laboured under a *mortal* disease at the time of the accident."

The second class, or that in which an interval elapses before the wound proves mortal, comprises a greater number of special cases. Before treating of these in detail, it is necessary to premise that, even when the interval between the injury and the fatal result is considerable, the death may be attributed to the injury without any misgiving ; for it may be such that no strength of constitution, and no care or skill, could avert a fatal termination. In fractures or dislocations of the spine, for instance, and in gun-shot wounds when the bullet lodges in the body, however long the fatal result may be postponed, the death is fairly attributable to the injury alone. But though, in cases of this kind, no doubt can exist either respecting the true cause of death or the guilt attaching to the act of violence, the lapse of time has, in most civilised countries, been taken into account ; and by the common law of

England, if the injured party survive one year and one day, the crime ceases to be murder; and English juries have sometimes shown a disposition to shorten this period very considerably.

Within this period of 366 days there is ample opportunity for some of the circumstances now to be specified to come into play.

1. A trifling wound or injury may prove fatal, from the injured part taking on an unhealthy character, such as scrofulous inflammation due to peculiarity of constitution, or erysipelatous inflammation from exposure to contagion.

2. To the same class of cases belong attacks of fatal tetanus or of delirium tremens from slight injuries, as well as rare instances of pyæmia from latent abscess brought into activity by a fall or blow, and fatal diseases of internal organs arising independent of, but soon after, the injury.

3. Another circumstance bearing on the question, Was the wound the cause of death? is the improper management of the wounded party: whether consisting in the neglect of medical assistance or of medical instructions; or in the resort to ignorant and unqualified practitioners; or in *mala praxis* on the part of a qualified medical attendant; * or in irregularities and reckless exposure to cold, fatigue, or fresh injury, or to intoxication, on the part of the patient himself.

Was the wound accidental, suicidal, or homicidal?— Accidental death is a common occurrence in crowds and in wrestlings and fights, when the deceased person falls or is thrown or struck against hard resisting objects, in which case an examination of the spot will help to determine the question.

There is always a probability of accident when a body is found in a dangerous situation, as at the foot of a precipice, or in a river with steep banks; and the probability is increased when the deceased is proved to have been drinking. In all doubtful cases the character of the injuries will go far to determine the class to which the death belongs. Bruises, fractures, and dislocations, for

---

* The following is the law relating to death from medical or surgical treatment with a view to cure, as defined by the Criminal Code Commission, sec. 173: " Every one who causes a bodily injury to any person from which death results, shall be deemed to kill that person, although the immediate cause of such death be treatment applied in good faith for the purpose of cure, even if such treatment was improper: Provided that if the injury was not in itself of a dangerous nature, and the improper treatment was the cause of the death, that shall be a defence to a charge of murder or manslaughter."

instance, are more consistent with the theory of death by accident than incised, punctured, or lacerated wounds.

The alternative of accident being excluded by the nature of the case, the original question is narrowed to this, Was the wound suicidal or homicidal?

As suicide is much more common than homicide, there is always a *primâ facie* probability in favour of suicide, especially in middle-aged persons; but this probability will be materially modified by such considerations as—**the place in which the body is found; the nature, seat, extent, and direction of the wound, and the number of wounds.**

Place where the body is found.—The finding of a corpse in a room with the windows and entrances fastened on the inside, is conclusive of suicide. The absence of the instrument of death is conclusive as to murder. So also, if the blood from a mortal wound has been washed from the body or floor, or is found on the feet or person of one affecting innocence (see case at p. 275, note), or if the body itself has been placed in a position inconsistent with the mode of death, or covered, or buried.

Nature of the wound.—Contused wounds are rarely suicidal, though attempts at self-destruction by knocking the head against the wall are not uncommon, especially among the insane. Severe contusions, therefore, are most probably homicidal, unless the body is lying near a height from which it might have fallen, or from which the deceased might have thrown himself. Incised wounds are as likely to be suicidal as homicidal, and it is not easy to infer from the character of the wound to which class it belongs. The cleanness and evenness of an incised wound would have indeed been thought to afford a probability in favour of homicide, but without sufficient reason, for a resolute suicide is more likely to have a steady hand than a murderer is to meet with no resistance; and some of the deepest and cleanest wounds of the throat are certainly suicidal.

In a few instances the shape of an incised wound helps to determine the question of suicide or homicide, by indicating the sort of instrument used, and the occupation of the murderer. Thus, a man with his throat cut from within to without, as butchers slaughter sheep, was found to have been murdered by a butcher; and in the case of a body divided in two by a cutting instrument passed into the fibro-cartilage uniting the third and fourth lumbar vertebræ, so as to divide the articulating processes transversely, as butchers cut through the spines of animals, a butcher was proved to have been the murderer (Orfila).

Seat of the wound.—If a wound is so situated that the instrument of death, when placed in the hand of the deceased, cannot be made to reach it, whether by the motion of the hand itself, or by that of the part injured, or by both jointly, it could not have been self-inflicted. Wounds on concealed parts, as within the labia and beneath the breast of the female, are in all probability homicidal. It must, however, be borne in mind that while murderers sometimes inflict injuries of a kind to appear as suicidal, many suicides are moved by very eccentric impulses.

Extent of the wound.—It has been thought that a suicide would not have courage or strength to inflict a very severe wound on himself; but experience is opposed to this view. Suicidal wounds of the throat, for instance, are usually deep and extensive; and nothing is more common than to read of the head being nearly severed from the body. But superficial wounds of the throat are among the most common forms of pretended suicide; and when two persons are found lying in the same room or place—the one severely wounded, perhaps dead, the other slightly, and alive—there is a strong presumption against the innocence of the survivor.

Direction of the wound.—Suicidal wounds generally follow the natural movement of the arm from left to right, and from above to below. But in the case of left-handed persons the direction would be reversed. Wounds of the throat, whether suicidal or homicidal, are, however, generally transverse. When persons of different statures fight, a wound inflicted by the taller man would pass from above downwards, and the reverse if given by the shorter, supposing both combatants to be standing. In wounds inflicted by a sword or by fire-arms, their direction and the orifices of entrance and exit should be noted.

Number of wounds. — The co-existence of several mortal wounds affords a presumption against suicide, but only a presumption; for after inflicting on themselves wounds necessarily mortal, suicides have retained strength and determination to inflict others. Thus, Orfila relates the case of a gentleman at Rouen found dead in his chamber, with two pistols lying, one near the body, the other on the bed, at some distance from it. He had shot himself in two places. One wound, apparently made while he was on the bed, had traversed the left side of the chest, breaking a rib before and behind, perforating the middle portion of the lung, and passing near the roots of the pulmonary veins. A large quantity of blood was extravasated in the chest. After inflicting on himself this serious injury, the deceased must have risen from the bed, walked to a closet to get another pistol, with which he produced a second wound that must have killed him instantly. The ball had entered the frontal bone, and after traversing the felt hemisphere of the brain, had lodged against the os occipitis. There was a doubt of this having been a deliberate suicide.

In a case reported in the " Times " of April 20th, 1872, Edward Mitchell, æt. 41, a sculptor, committed suicide by inflicting wounds in the breast by means of a graving tool, 6 or 7 inches long and of a bayonet shape, and afterwards throwing himself from the window of the fourth storey of a house. He had stabbed himself first in the left ventricle, and secondly in the right, in which the instrument remained deeply fixed. The handle of the instrument had come off with the violence, and was laid by the deceased on the mantelpiece. The suicide then went from the third to the fourth storey and threw himself from the window; on the instrument being removed, he became sensible, spoke, and lived for three hours.

Watson gives a case of suicide in which no less than ten wounds were inflicted on the throat.

As most of the probabilities just established may lead to error if too implicitly relied upon, we have to be on our guard against false inferences from circumstances purely accidental, as well as from arrangements made to deceive us.

Nor is it always safe to assume that a severe injury actually inflicted by another is the real cause of death; for, as in a case related by Walberg, a death occurring during a chastisement may, on examination, be found to have been due to poison.

The circumstantial evidence in death by wounds is of great inportance. (See " Persons found Dead," p. 273.) Sellis, a servant of the Duke of Cumberland, afterwards King of Hanover, was found dead on his bed with his throat cut, while his master, severely wounded in the head and hand, was under the care of Sir Everard Home. The Duke stated that he was roused from sleep by a blow on the head, followed by several others, one of which caused an immense effusion of blood; that he leaped out of bed, and followed his assailant, who repeatedly struck at him, and would doubtless have murdered him, but that the doors protected his person from some of the blows. Every part of this statement was confirmed by the circumstantial evidence. The coloured drapery at the head of the Duke's bed was sprinkled with blood; there were traces of blood on the passages and staircase, and on the doors of all the State apartments; and Sellis's coat was found on a chair out of reach of blood from his bed, but with the sleeve sprinkled from shoulder to wrist "with blood, quite dry, and evidently from a wounded artery."

Lord William Russell, the victim of Courvoisier, was found dead in bed with his throat cut; the instrument of death did not lie near the body, and a napkin was placed over the face. A woman of the name of Norkott was found dead in bed with her throat cut, and on her *left hand* a bloody mark of a *left hand*. In both these cases the evidence of murder was complete.

There are still other questions to be considered—as, for instance, whether a given wound is dangerous to life, and of many wounds, which was mortal. It may also be important to know how long the wounded person survived the injury, and to fix the point of time at which a wound was inflicted.

Is the wound dangerous to life?—It is easy to answer this question in the case of injuries to large blood-vessels and important viscera, less easy in the case of injuries which affect life rather by their extent than the importance of the parts implicated; for while, on the one hand, slight injuries to unimportant parts may, in peculiar states of constitution, prove fatal, on the other, men may recover from injuries the most severe and extensive, as in the well-known case of Mr. Tipper, pinned against a stable-door by the shaft of a gig traversing the chest.

The danger attending injuries of the several important parts of the body will be found discussed under the next heading.

Of many wounds, which was mortal?—It is easy to understand how this question may become important. A mortal struggle may begin with blows and end with the use of a stabbing or cutting instrument; and the crime would have a very different aspect according as the death was attributable to the blows or to the stabs or cuts. The question is of so general a nature that it must suffice to indicate its importance.

How long did the wounded person survive?—This

question, too, may evidently assume importance, especially in connection with the amount of exertion possible after severe injuries. It involves many details, and must be reserved for the next division.

When was the wound inflicted?—This question may arise either during life or after death. During life the question must be answered, in the case of contused wounds, by the extent of the ecchymosis and the colour it assumes; in the cases of incised and punctured wounds, by the state of the divided parts, whether they are filled with extravasated blood or not; and whether the edges are swollen, and the surrounding skin inflamed. After death the question either resolves itself into the simple inquiry, how long has the deceased been dead? or into the double question of the date of the death and the length of time that the deceased survived. The presence or absence of animal heat, of cadaveric rigidity, and of putrefaction, and the progress which putrefaction may have made, must be taken into account. These changes take place, as already observed (p. 284), with very different degrees of rapidity in different subjects, so as to oblige us to speak of the time they occupy with caution and reserve.

V. WOUNDS AS THEY AFFECT THE SEVERAL PARTS OF THE BODY.

Some of the questions which have been indicated as important in the previous division will be examined in detail in this.

Wounds of the head.—Injuries to the scalp are more important than those of the integuments of other parts, on account of the peculiar tendency of the skin itself to take on the erysipelatous inflammation; the quantity of loose areolar tissue intervening between the tendon of the occipito-frontalis and the periosteum, which is very liable to become the seat of diffuse inflammation, and the relation of the tendon to this lax tissue, preventing, as it does, the escape of effused products. Punctured and contused wounds of the scalp are dangerous on account of the inflammation they set up in this tissue, and the want of free exit for the discharges; but extensive lacerated wounds which do not involve the periosteum are rarely serious, inasmuch as they afford free passage to the products of inflammation.

Fractures of the skull are not of themselves more important than those of other bones, but for the fact that the injury that occasions the fracture also produces concussion or other injury to the brain or its membranes. A blow on the skull, it should be observed, does not always fracture the bone on which it alights, but may produce a counter-fracture at an opposite part of the skull—fracture by a counter-stroke. A severe blow or fall on the vertex of the head, for instance, will often occasion a fracture at the base.

The danger attending injuries to the skull varies with the thickness of the part struck. A blow on the temple would produce greater injury than one of equal force applied to other parts; the thinness of the orbital plate and of the cribriform plate of the ethmoid bone, exposes the brain to serious injury from thrusts with pointed instruments.

Injuries of the brain may be classified under the heads of **Concussion** or commotion; **Contusion, Compression, Wounds, Inflammation** and its consequences (encephalitis and meningo-encephalitis).

Concussion, or commotion.—This is a term applied to the assemblage of symptoms resulting from a violent jar to the nerve centres, such as may be caused by a direct blow on the head, or communicated to it through the spine—as by a fall on the buttocks.

The symptoms occur immediately on receipt of the blow, and vary in intensity and duration. Consciousness is lost, there is complete muscular relaxation, the face is pale, the pupils dilated and respond to light imperfectly if at all, the pulse is feeble and frequent, and the respiration superficial or irregular. Nausea and vomiting usually occur as the patient begins to recover. In some cases these symptoms are transient—a momentary stun—but in others they last some hours, or death may take place without reaction; or the patient may recover from the concussion, die from effusion with compression, or from inflammation and its consequences.

The exact pathology of concussion has been much discussed, but it is possible for fatal concussion to occur without any other marked appearances beyond general venous congestion.

Contusion.—Contusion is not unfrequently caused by the same injury which causes concussion. It is characterised by the appearance at the seat of injury, or on the opposite side, or at the base of the brain, of scattered punctiform hæmorrhages, situated superficially, or, it may be, in the substance of the brain.*

* See Duret : " Sur Traumatismes Cérébraux." Thèse, 1878.

In such cases, in addition to the symptoms characteristic of concussion, we may have superadded symptoms indicative of localised lesions in the form of paralysis or convulsions.

Contusion is very apt to be followed by hæmorrhagic effusion of considerable amount, leading to compression ; or by inflammation.

Compression of the brain.—This may result from depressed fracture of the skull, and the symptoms may remain for a long period, and be immediately relieved by elevation of the depressed bone.

Compression may also result from effusion of blood on the surface or in the substance of the brain, or from the products of inflammation set up by a cranial injury.

Compression is a common sequence of concussion with contusion, and it is not always easy to determine whether we have to deal with concussion merely, or with concussion and compression.

Very often, however, the individual recovers from concussion, and after an hour or two begins to complain of pain in the head, noises in the ears, giddiness, sickness, confusion of ideas, and weariness ; gradually passing into stupor and coma, with complete loss of consciousness, dilated or unequal pupils, stertorous breathing and slow pulse.   Convulsions also may occur.

These symptoms are due to the more copious effusion of blood from the ruptured vessels during the reaction which takes place after the first shock of the concussion ; but if the symptoms of compression do not come on for several days after the concussion, we cannot attribute them to hæmorrhage.

Rapid and fatal hæmorrhage is specially apt to occur from fracture of the anterior inferior angle of the parietal bone and rupture of the middle meningeal artery, and consequent effusion between the dura mater and the skull.   Or the effusion is on the surface of the brain from rupture of the vessels of the pia mater. But effusion of blood from cranial injury may also take place (though rarely) in the interior.

In compression due to depressed bone the cause of death is obvious ; but when it arises from effusion following injury, it may be alleged that the effusion and consequent fatal results were due, not to the injury itself, but to some concomitant circumstance. Thus, if in the course of a struggle a man is thrown down or struck, and dies soon after with symptoms of compression, and an effusion of blood has taken place, this may be attributed to the excitement of the contest, and not to the injury itself; and this is the more likely to be the case if the deceased was given to habits of intoxication, or was by age or disease predisposed to apoplexy.

In such cases careful search must be made for indications of disease of the blood-vessels, such as atheroma or miliary aneurisms, disease of the kidneys, hypertrophy of the heart, in all of which conditions cerebral hæmorrhage is specially apt to occur. Should none of these conditions be met with, if the individual is young, and the effusion is from the middle meningeal or on the surface of the brain, death is to be attributed to the cranial injury. If the signs of disease co-exist with those of the cranial injury, probably both factors may have been at work, and there will be room for difference of opinion.

Wounds.—Wounds of the brain are very variable in their effects. While fatal effusion or inflammation may result from comparatively slight wounds, on the other hand, recovery may take place, especially in the young, from the most extensive laceration and loss of substance, and with comparatively little effect on the mental and bodily powers.

Many such cases are recorded in the works of Paré, Wiseman, and modern surgical writers. A well-known case is the American crow-bar case, in which recovery took place after the passage of an iron bar through the left side of the frontal lobe.* Wounds may be made in the frontal, occipital, or tempero-sphenoidal lobes without producing paralytic symptoms; but if the convolutions bounding the fissure of Rolando are affected, general or partial paralysis of the opposite side ensues according to the extent and position of the lesion.† Aphasia has resulted from traumatic lesions of the left hemisphere in the region known as Broca's convolution. When a bullet or other missile lodges in the brain, an interval of several days may elapse before symptoms of inflammation show themselves; the patient meanwhile lying free from suffering, but showing by some such symptoms as aphasia that the function of some part of the brain has been destroyed.

Inflammation.—Inflammation of the brain (encephalitis) and its membranes (meningitis) is a very common result of injuries of the head, whether the skull be fractured or not—most frequently

* See Ferrier: "The Localisation of Cerebral Disease," 1878.
† On this, see Ferrier, *op. cit.*

in the former case. It is also a very insidious sequela, often showing itself many days or even weeks after the receipt of the injury. Most commonly after a week or ten days the symptoms make their appearance, during which interval the patient may apparently have quite recovered. The result may be diffuse inflammation and suppuration, or a large cerebral abscess may form, leading to death with all the symptoms of compression. A very instructive case of cerebral abscess, resulting from a blow on the head without fracture of the skull, has been put on record by Dr. Burney Yeo.* No distinct symptoms pointing to cerebral lesion showed themselves for more than six weeks after receipt of the injury, and death did not ensue for three weeks after they were fairly developed.

Injuries of the head, therefore, have this peculiarity, that at first they often seem of little consequence, but after an interval, which is often considerable, dangerous symptoms arise and end fatally. During this interval a patient may be neglected or mismanaged, or may so misconduct himself as materially to affect the question—Was the injury the cause of death? Such injuries, even if they do not prove fatal, not unfrequently cause epilepsy, paralysis, or even insanity, at a more or less distant date.

Injuries of the spinal cord.—The spinal cord is liable to the same affections as the brain, and from similar causes: the two are often affected together by the same injury. We may have concussion or commotion from violent blows on the back, or jars; compression from the effusion of blood or by dislocated or fractured vertebræ; wounds; and local or general meningitis and myelitis.

The effect of lesions of the spinal cord varies with their seat. Injuries of the medulla oblongata and upper part of the spinal cord, such as occur from dislocation of the neck or fracture of the cervical vertebræ, are instantly fatal, by affecting the centres of circulation and respiration. In general, if the injury is below the origin of the phrenic nerve, but above the origin of the brachial plexus, paralysis of all the limbs and trunk ensues—an injury which may be fatal in a few hours, or after the lapse of many weeks, or months, or even years. In the case of John Carter, of Coggeshall, in Essex, displacement of the last three cervical vertebræ, with pressure on the cord opposite the seventh vertebra, did not prove fatal for fourteen years.

* *Brit. Med. Journ.*, June 7 and 14, 1879.

When the cord is injured in the dorsal or lumbar region there is paralysis or impairment of motion and sensation below the seat of injury, with loss of control over the sphincters.

Such injuries would be speedily fatal but for constant attention and nursing, but with these aids life may be prolonged for many years.

Of great importance in a medico-legal point of view are the effects of spinal concussion, more particularly in connection with railway accidents, a fertile source of litigation.*

In some cases death results from general spinal concussion; in others, a temporary paraplegia, with pains in the limbs, ensues, from which the individual may entirely recover in the course of a day or two. On the other hand, the recovery may only be partial, and the patient suffers from weakness, pains, and abnormal sensations in the limbs, with wasting of the muscles and tenderness on percussion of the spine, for a long period subsequently, though he may eventually recover.

In other cases the symptoms do not show themselves immediately on receipt of the injury, but make their appearance often weeks or months afterwards, and are attributed to slowly progressive degeneration in the cord and membranes.

The patient becomes exceedingly emotional and hysterical, irritable and sleepless, and incapable of mental exertion. Sight becomes impaired. The limbs are weak and the gait unsteady or ataxic. The back is stiff and painful on movement or percussion; numbness and perverted sensations are complained of in the limbs; but there is seldom complete paralysis either of motion or sensation. The nutrition of the muscles also suffers, and they often lose their contractility. The bladder is weak and the sexual powers are greatly impaired or lost. There is general impairment of nutrition, coldness of the extremities, and other signs of general prostration.

This assemblage of symptoms is said to be characteristic of "railway spine," but as many of them are of a purely subjective character, and the individuals often wilfully simulate or exaggerate symptoms, the utmost caution is necessary, and special knowledge of nervous diseases is required, in order correctly to appreciate the real amount of injury sustained. So long, however, as the present

* On this subject, see Erichsen "On Concussion of the Spine," 1875; Erb on "Diseases of the Spinal Cord," Ziemssen's "Cyclopædia."

system of examining injuries and awarding damages prevails, we may continue to expect the not very edifying conflicts of opinion among medical witnesses in courts of law.

Wounds of the face.—These not only occasion disfigurement, but, in consequence of the free distribution of important nerves, still more grave inconvenience. From the near proximity of the principal features to the brain, there is also a risk of injury to that organ, as well as of inflammation extending from the seat of the wound.

Wounds of the throat.—These are the cause of death in a great majority of suicides, and sometimes a murderer inflicts a wound on the same part, hoping that his victim will be supposed to have committed suicide. The degree of danger depends on the parts implicated; wounds of the anterior part of the throat being less dangerous than those of the side of the neck; those of the lower part less so than those of the upper. A division of the carotid artery is almost necessarily fatal, and that of the internal jugular vein attended with great danger from hæmorrhage, from the introduction of air into the circulation, and from phlebitis. Wounds of the larynx or trachea are attended with comparatively little danger, those of the trachea being less important than those of the larynx.

The question, Was the wound the cause of death? is easily answered; but the question, Was the wound suicidal or homicidal? not so readily. There is also a question of considerable interest relating to these wounds—namely, What amount of voluntary motion is possible after the receipt of a severe wound?

These questions of suicide or homicide, and of the amount of voluntary motion possible after a severe wound in the throat, were raised in the case of Captain Wright, who shared the captivity of Sir Sydney Smith and his celebrated escape from the Temple, and who had the misfortune to be taken a second time and imprisoned in the same place. He was found dead in his bed with his throat cut, and a razor closed in his right hand. There was an extensive transverse wound on the anterior and superior parts of the throat, above the hyoid bone, cutting through the skin, the muscles, the windpipe, the gullet, and the blood-vessels, and penetrating to the cervical vertebræ. The circumstances of the case are involved in so much mystery that it is impossible to determine by the evidence collected with great pains by Sir Sydney Smith, whether Wright really committed suicide or not; but that the mere fact of the razor being found closed in his hand does not militate very strongly against the supposition of suicide is shown by the cases that follow. In September 1838, an officer in the army was found dead, with the head nearly severed from the body, and there was no doubt that the act was suicidal; yet the razor had been put on the dressing-table. A madman, after inflicting a severe wound on his throat, had time to struggle with the maid-servant before he fell down dead. In October 1833, a man cut his throat with a razor while walking along Oxford Street, dividing the carotid artery and several of its branches, the jugular vein on one side, and the trachea; yet he was seen to hold a handkerchief to his neck, and run four yards before he fell dead on the pavement. He held the razor firmly grasped in his hand.

In the remarkable case of Mary Green, murdered in 1832 by John Danks, the confession of the culprit, and the circumstantial evidence coincided to prove that, after a wound which divided *the trunk of the carotid artery, and all the principal branches of the external carotid, with the jugulars,* she must have risen from the ground, run a distance of *twenty-three yards,* and climbed over a low gate. It took from fifteen to twenty seconds to run from the spot on which the murder was committed to that on which the body was found.

Wounds of the chest.—Incised wounds of the walls of the chest are not dangerous; but severe blows often prove fatal by the shock they occasion, or by fracturing the bones, and causing rupture of the viscera, leading to hæmorrhage or inflammation. Such injuries occur in prize-fights, in falls from great heights, and from heavy objects crushing the chest. Penetrating wounds of the chest can scarcely fail to injure some important organ, occasioning thereby fatal hæmorrhage or severe subsequent inflammation; but cases are recorded of sword and gun-shot wounds traversing the chest without causing any bad symptoms; and most of the cases of injury to the chest that were under Wiseman's care after the battle of Dunbar seem to have recovered.

Wounds of the lungs.—Hæmorrhage is the immediate consequence of these injuries. The blood may be discharged by the wound or by expectoration, or it may accumulate in the cavity of the pleura, causing great difficulty of breathing. When the large vessels are wounded, the hæmorrhage is copious and speedily fatal.

Injuries to the substance of the lung itself are not necessarily fatal, for patients have recovered after removal of a portion of the lung; and in rare instances foreign bodies, such as bullets, have remained in the lungs for years, enclosed in cysts. Inflammation is a common consequence of these wounds, especially when foreign substances are introduced, as happens in injuries with fire-arms. Cases of wounds of the lungs require careful management and long-continued rest. Emphysema is a familiar effect of these wounds, but when judiciously treated does not materially increase the danger.

Wounds of the heart.—Penetrating wounds of the heart are speedily fatal from hæmorrhage, unless they pass so obliquely through the walls that the flap acts like a valve, or a foreign body happen to plug the orifice, when death may be delayed for some hours, or even days. Wounds of the base prove more speedily fatal than those of the apex, and superficial wounds that divide the nutrient vessels less promptly than such as penetrate its cavities. John Bell gives the case of a soldier in whom the apex of the heart was cut with the point of a long and slender sword; and yet this man lived twelve hours, during which time the heart had at every stroke been losing a small quantity of blood, till it entirely filled the chest and suffocated him. Another man was wounded with a sword, the point of which cut the coronary artery; but it was two hours before the pericardium filled with blood, and then, after a great anxiety, the patient died. In very rare instances, when the wound does not prove fatal by hæmorrhage, complete recovery takes place; as in a case related by Fournier, and authenticated by M. Mansen, chief surgeon to the hospital at Orleans, of a patient who died six years after receiving a gun-shot wound, from disease unconnected with it, when the ball was found embedded in the heart. MM. Olliver and Sanson have collected a number of cases of penetrating wounds of the heart, with a view of determining the average period at which they prove fatal. Out of twenty-nine cases of wounds of the cavities only two were fatal within forty-eight hours; in the remainder, death took place in periods varying from four to twenty-eight days.[*]

Wounds of the aorta and pulmonary artery are

---

[*] " Dict. des Sciences Médicales," art. *Cas rares.*

necessarily fatal; but patients have lived a few days after small punctured wounds even of the aorta.

Wounds of the œsophagus and thoracic duct.—Such injuries are necessarily rare, from the great depth at which these parts lie. They are dangerous from the extravasation of their contents. Orifila records a recovery from a bayonet-wound of the œsophagus.

Wounds of the diaphragm.—Punctured wounds of this part do not appear to be attended with great danger, unless they involve injury to the parts above or below. Fatal hernia of the stomach or lung may result. Death may take place after a long interval from the protrusion of the viscera of the abdomen into the chest, and consequent functional disturbance. Rupture of the diaphragm from severe blows or falls is in most cases attended by nervous shock and sudden death.

Wounds of the abdomen.—Incised wounds of the abdominal walls may prove fatal by dividing the epigastric artery. In wounds of the tendons, as in scalp wounds, danger may arise from the accumulation of matter. Ventral hernia is a remote consequence of wounds of the abdominal walls. Severe blows may prove fatal by shock, hæmorrhage from ruptured viscera, or inflammation. The liver and spleen are the organs most liable to rupture.

Wounds of the liver.—Deep penetrating wounds of this organ usually prove fatal by dividing the large vessels, but sometimes by giving rise to inflammation; and wounds of the gall-bladder by causing effusion of bile, and consequent peritoneal inflammation.

Wounds of the spleen.—Deep wounds are fatal by hæmorrhage; but superficial wounds are not always mortal. Rupture of the spleen by blows is fatal, according to the amount of injury, in from a few hours to several days. In a convalescent patient a kick over an enlarged and extremely soft spleen caused the effusion of several ounces of blood, and death in a few minutes.*

Wounds of the stomach.—These kill by shock, by hæmorrage from the large vessels, by extravasation of the contents and consequent peritoneal inflammation, and by inflammation of the viscus itself. But they are not always fatal, and many cases of recovery are recorded, even when the wound was extensive, and the stomach distended with food.

* Robert Williams: "Elements of Medicine," vol. ii. p. 470.

Wounds of the intestines.—These prove fatal, like those of the stomach by hæmorrhage, by discharge of the contents and consequent peritonitis, or by inflammation. The danger is great in the small intestines, and greatest in the duodenum, from the fluid state of their contents and greater risk of extravasation. Wounds of the intestines sometimes heal by the effusion and organisation of coagulable lymph.

Wounds of the kidneys.—Penetrating wounds of the kidneys may cause fatal hæmorrhage, extravasation of urine, or inflammation. If the urine can be prevented from flowing into the peritoneal cavity, recovery may take place.

Wounds of the bladder, especially when the organ is distended, prove fatal by extravasation of urine into the abdominal cavity or cellular tissue, and consequent inflammation, of the peritoneum. After rupture of the bladder the sufferer may walk some distance; but the accident is apt to prove ultimately though not speedily fatal, though recovery may occur if the wound is treated surgically.

Wounds of the genital organs.—Removal of the penis, if not fatal by hæmorrhage, is not dangerous; but an incised wound of the urethra entails the risk of extravasation of urine and fatal sloughing. The removal of the testicles is attended with less danger than a contusion, which sometimes proves fatal by shock. Wounds of the spermatic cord occasion dangerous hæmorrhage. The complete removal of all the parts of generation of the male may lead to no bad result. Deep wounds of the labia of the female are dangerous from hæmorrhage. Fatal injuries have been inflicted on the uterus, bladder, or rectum, or on the large vessels of the pelvis, by instruments introduced into the vagina.

Consult Watson's "Medico-legal Treatise on Homicide."

VI. DETECTION OF BLOOD-STAINS, HAIR, &c.

The medical jurist may have to examine red spots supposed to be caused by blood on wearing apparel, on cutting instruments, on floors or furniture, or wherever they may have fallen; also, in some cases to examine watery solutions of blood; and he may be asked to distinguish the blood of man from that of animals, and to assign the source whence it flowed.

When the blood-spot is recent and the quantity large, it presents highly characteristic appearances, and yields a solution of a peculiar colour, readily distinguished from all other red fluids by its chemical, microscopical, and spectroscopical properties. But when the spots are not recent, and the quantity of blood is small, great care is needed in the work of identification; the blood-colouring matter may have been changed into methæmoglobin or into hæmatin; or rendered insoluble by heat or by chemical agents in the material on which the stain is present.

We will first describe these tests, and then show their application to the detection of stains.

i. **Chemical tests.**—The colouring matter of the blood is completely soluble in cold water, and yields a red solution, which is *coagulated by heat*, and changed to a dirty slate colour. The addition of *liquor potassæ* dissolves the clot, and yields a solution, dark green by transmitted, and red by reflected light. The coagulum reappears on the addition of nitric acid. The blood solution has also the characteristic property of not being changed in colour by the addition of a small quantity of *liquor ammoniæ*. No other red solutions have these two characters. The red, pink, or scarlet infusions of flowers and roots, and the juices of fruits, are changed to green or violet by ammonia, and cochineal to crimson. The red solution of the thiocyanide (sulphocyanide) of iron yields with the same reagent a precipitate of oxide of iron; and the pink solution of permanganate of potassium is changed to blue. Chlorine water turns the blood solution at first slightly green, then discolours it, and produces, especially on warming a flocculent white precipitate.

Blood solutions yield a red precipitate, to *infusion of tannin* or *tincture of galls;* but red colouring matters, due to salts of iron, a dark blue precipitate. *Acetate of zinc*, in presence of ammonia, throws down a flocculent reddish precipitate (Gunning).

A solution of *tungstate of sodium,* acidulated with acetic or phosphoric acid, gives a red precipitate, soluble in ammonia, forming a dichroic, greenish-red fluid, again precipitated by acids. The precipitate, when fused with soda and a little nitre, leaves an insoluble residue of oxide of iron (Sonnenschein).

Ozonic or guiacum test. — The blood-solution possesses the property of transferring ozone from substances that contain it (peroxide of hydrogen, ozonic ether, or oil of turpentine) to ozone reagents, such as tincture of guaiacum, which are oxidized and change colour. If to a solution of the colouring matter of the blood a few drops of tincture of guaiacum* are added, and then a few drops of solution of peroxide of hydrogen, a rich, sapphire-blue colour results. This test is directly applicable to stains on linen, which, when moistened with tincture of guaiacum, and then with peroxide of hydrogen solution, assume a blue colour. This test, though very delicate, is not quite conclusive, as certain other substances give a similar reaction with guaiacum.

Hæmin test.—Of all the tests for the colouring matter of blood this is the most certain. But as there are certain conditions in which it fails, such failure must not be taken to prove the absence of blood. If the test succeeds, it is conclusive of its presence. To apply this test, we use the blood solution evaporated to dryness, or a small portion of dried blood from a stain, or the precipitate caused by tannin or acetate of zinc. The dried residue of the solution in a watch-glass, or a portion of dried blood on a microscope slide, is covered with glacial acetic acid, a crystal of chloride of sodium added, and then carefully heated to boiling over a spirit-lamp. It is well to add the acid more than once, especially

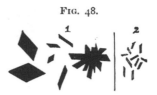

FIG. 48.

× 300 Diameters.   × 150.

if a slide is used. On allowing the mass to cool, the microscope reveals, mixed with crystals of chloride and acetate of sodium, immense numbers of dark-brown rhombic prisms of hæmin, as in fig. 48, after Virchow, in which (1) shows large crystals, and (2) small crystals from a minute recent spot of sheep's blood. They vary much in size according to the rate of crystallisation.

These crystals are a compound of hydrochloric acid with hæmatin, which is one of the products of the decomposition of hæmoglobin. They are known as *Teichmann's crystals.*

If the stain has been dissolved in a solution of common salt (1 in 200), it is not necessary to add the chloride of sodium.

2. **Spectroscopic test.**—Solutions of the colouring matter of the blood, examined by the spectroscope, give a spectrum characterised by the presence of definite absorption bands. A bright source of artificial light is preferable to daylight, as otherwise the presence of Frauenhofer's lines may be embarrassing; the position of the D line can at once easily be ascertained by placing in a flame a

* Made from the interior of a piece of resin, and diluted to a brownish yellow tint.

platinum wire previously dipped in a sodium solution. If the blood solution is too concentrated, only the red end of the spectrum is visible. When of the right degree of concentration, two dark absorption bands are seen in the green between the lines D and E. The first absorption band (*i.e.* from the left) is narrower and more sharply defined than the second, which is separated from it by a

FIG. 49.*

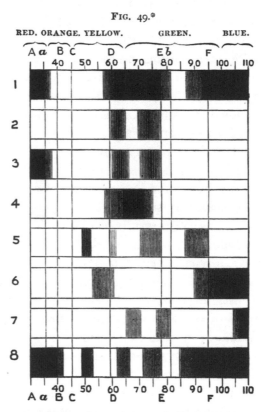

1. Oxyhæmoglobin, 0·8 per cent. 2. Oxyhæmoglobin, 0·18 per cent. 3. Carbonic oxide hæmoglobin. 4. Reduced hæmoglobin. 5. Hæmatin in alcohol with sulphuric acid. 6. Hæmatin in alkaline solution. 7. Reduced hæmatin. 8. Methæmoglobin. (Altered from Landois and Stirling.)

green interspace. In very dilute solutions the second is the first to disappear. The spectrum, with the two absorption bands, is that of oxidized hæmoglobin (oxyhæmoglobin) (2, fig. 49). When a reducing agent is added to the solution, such as ammonium or sodium sulphide, or a solution of ferrous sulphate acidified with tartaric acid to prevent precipitation by alkalies, the two bands disappear ; and in their stead one only is seen, dark in the middle,

* See Frontispiece.

and with washed-out edges, occupying what was the green inter-space between the two bands of oxidised hæmoglobin. This is the spectrum of reduced hæmoglobin (4, Fig. 49).* By shaking the solution with air it is again re-oxidised, and gives the spectrum with the two lines as before.

A red solution possessed of the above characters can only be a solution of blood-colouring matter. Other red solutions, such as carmine and alkanet, give spectra which, on careless inspection, might be mistaken for solutions of hæmoglobin; but their bands do not occupy exactly the same position in the spectrum, nor are they capable of reduction and re-oxidation in the manner described. The reduction test should therefore always be had recourse to in determining by the spectroscope whether a given solution is a blood solution or not. Hæmoglobin, on the other hand, is liable to undergo decomposition spontaneously and under the influence of various reagents, and the spectrum undergoes corresponding alterations. In stains a few weeks old, hæmoglobin becomes changed into methæmoglobin, which is readily dissolved out by water. This body gives a spectrum (8, in Fig. 49)† in which the red and blue are in great part cut off, and one band appears between C and D, and two bands in the green between D and E are seen. If ammonia be added, the spectrum shows two bands like oxyhæmo-globin; the first band, however, extending more into the red. If the solution be deoxidised by ammonium sulphide, the spectrum of reduced hæmoglobin is seen (4, in Fig. 49), from which that of oxyhæmoglobin is readily obtainable. By long exposure to the air, or under the influence of acids and alkalies, hæmoglobin is decomposed into a brown colouring matter, hæmatin, and a proteid substance. Thus, when acetic acid is added to a solution of hæmo-globin, the solution becomes brown from the formation of hæmatin, and if the turbid fluid be shaken with ether, a clear ethereal solution will be obtained, which when examined with the spectro-scope, shows a characteristic absorption band coinciding nearly with Frauenhofer's line C in the confines of the red and orange (5, Fig. 49).‡ Similarly, alkalies split up hæmoglobin into hæmatin and a proteid substance. In this case the hæmatin band is broader, and is situated lower down the spectrum nearer the line D, while the blue end of the spectrum is much obscured (6, Fig. 49).§

* See frontispiece, Fig. 5.   † Ibid., Fig. 9.
‡ Ibid., Fig. 6.   § Ibid., Fig. 7.

2 B

This alkaline hæmatin possesses the property of being reducible like hæmoglobin, and again oxidisable. The spectrum of reduced hæmatin is characterised by two well-defined absorption bands, similar to those of oxyhæmoglobin, but situated lower down nearer the blue (7, Fig. 49).

In applying the spectroscopic test for blood, the ordinary spectroscope may be used if the quantity is comparatively large. The colouring power of hæmoglobin is very intense, 1 in 4500 of water giving the absorption bands in the ordinary spectroscope. If the quantity is minute—such as may be got from a small stain— Sorby and Browning's micro-spectroscope should be employed in the investigation (Fig. 50). This consists of an instrument which can be substituted for the eyepiece of the microscope, and contains the requisite prismatic arrangements for placing side by side a spectrum of the object on the stage, and (by the slide slit) a second beam of light from any object whose spectrum it is desired to compare with that of the object on the stage. By means of focussing arrangements, with which the apparatus is supplied, the light can be readily adjusted, and the spectra and absorption bands accurately defined.*

FIG. 50.

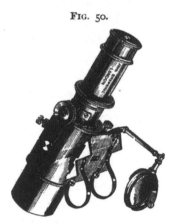

By means of this instrument the spectrum of hæmoglobin may be obtained from a few blood corpuscles.

In dealing with very weak solutions of the colouring matter of the blood, it is necessary to obtain a certain depth of colour before the absorption bands become visible. For this purpose the cells invented by Mr. Sorby are admirably adapted. One form consists of a piece of barometer tubing about an inch in length, which is soldered on to a glass slide. By proper focussing and arrangement of the diaphragm, the light is made to traverse the whole column of the fluid, and thus with a very slightly coloured solution a sufficient degree of concentration is obtained. The other form is a wedge-shaped microscopical cell. When closed with a covering of glass, a wedge-shaped body of fluid is obtained, and the thick or thin edge placed in front of the objective, as required. These cells

* Sorby : "Proc. Roy. Soc.," vol. xv. ; and various other memoirs.

also allow of the addition of reducing agents to the solution, so that all the spectroscopic reactions can be studied with excessively small quantities. The spectroscopic test for blood colouring matter exceeds in delicacy all others.

3. **Microscopical characters.**—Blood is recognised under the microscope by the presence of the red (and white) corpuscles. The red corpuscles are highly characteristic. Their microscopic characters require to be well studied, inasmuch as circular forms are very commonly met with, as in the oil-globules of milk, the spores of yeast, and many crystalloids, organic and inorganic. The appearance of the globules in mammalia is shown in plan and section, largely magnified, in the figure (Fig. 51), after Gulliver. They have also been depicted in plan as a circular disc with shaded centre; in section as a biconcave lens. But their appearance differs with the power of the microscope, the light, and the focus. When

FIG. 51.

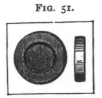

FIG. 52.

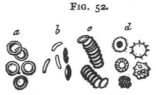

Magnified 400 diameters

viewed by transmitted light, they appear, when out of focus, as convex discs with faint outlines; as we approach the true focus, the outline becomes dark and distinct; and when quite in focus, they seem to have a dark inner margin, a slight shaded depression, or a dark central shadow. Similar changes take place when the mirror is slowly moved, so as to place the object under a succession of brighter and dimmer lights. The observer should provide himself with a standard specimen of human blood globules with which to compare, for form and size, that which happens to be under investigation. The figure (Fig. 52) shows the blood corpuscles as isolated discs—(a) in plan; (b) in profile; (c) aggregated like piles of coin; (d) variously contracted and crimped by the exudation of their contents. Under the influence of water the red corpuscles swell up and become globular, lose their colour, and eventually disappear. Solutions denser than the blood plasma cause them to shrivel and assume irregular forms. The white corpuscles are fewer in number, but somewhat larger in size. They have a granular aspect, and contain one or more nuclei.

Examination of blood-stains.—Blood-stains on linen.—
Before applying the tests, note should be made of the article of
dress and the position and number of the stains; whether the
stains are on the inside or outside of the garment; and, if one or
more articles of dress are stained, whether they are in a corresponding part.

Blood-stains have certain characters recognisable without extraneous aid. A spot of blood not disturbed by contact or friction
feels like thick gum or starch. Small spots are circular, large
spots approach that form; large and small alike have a defined
and abrupt margin.

Arterial blood has a bright red colour, and venous blood a dark
or purple hue, but it becomes arterial on exposure to the air. After
the lapse of a few hours both kinds of blood lose their bright colour
and assume a reddish-brown hue, which may remain unchanged
for years. When it has assumed this colour we cannot give any
opinion as to its age.*

Certain of the above-mentioned tests are at once applicable to
the stains before proceeding to apply others. A small stain or part
of a stain, if only one exist, may be cut out and tested with liquor
ammoniæ. This will at once distinguish blood from vegetable
colouring matters. To a similar fragment (a single fibre will
suffice) let a drop of tincture of guaiacum and a drop of peroxide
of hydrogen be added on a slide. If blood-colouring matter is
present, a sapphire blue colour will result. If the stain is dry, this
reaction does not take place till the texture has become moistened.
The other tests, with the exception of the hæmin test, which is perhaps more conveniently applied before solution, require the solution
of the colouring matter. A small scraping of the stain is to be laid
on a slide, a crystal of chloride of sodium added, and then boiled
with glacial acetic acid in the manner before described. As already
stated, the production of hæmin crystals is the best proof of the
existence of blood. If we use a solution of the stain, it is best
made in a solution of common salt (1 in 200). The stain is to be
cut out and suspended by a thread in a test-tube or watch-glass
containing a small quantity of the saline solution. A recent stain

* Dr. Pfaff has suggested a solution of arsenious acid (gr. j. to ℨij) as a blood
solvent and means of ascertaining the age of a stain. He thought that he could
fix the age by the quicker or slower solution of the colouring matter. His own
loose statements as to the time required sufficiently condemn his not very
promising proposal.

so treated generally yields a reddish or reddish-brown solution, the colour being more intense in the deeper strata. An old stain gives up its colour very slowly and imperfectly, the process taking many hours. The solution may be aided by tearing the fibres of the cloth and by agitation. If the stain is very old, all the colouring matter will have become converted into hæmatin. It will not dissolve in water, but it may be dissolved out more or less completely by ammonia. If the colouring matter is insoluble in water or simple ammonia, it must be treated with ammonia (1 part) and rectified spirit (5 parts). If it be still difficult to dissolve, heat the solution. This solution will give the spectrum of alkaline hæmatin; and if the bands are very indistinct, it must be treated with ammonium sulphide, after which the two bands of reduced hæmatin are plainly visible (MacMunn).*

The cloth from which the solution has been made may be examined with the microscope for the presence of adherent blood corpuscles and threads of insoluble fibrin (see Fig. 53) which may remain after the colouring matter has been dissolved.

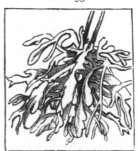

FIG. 53.

After Gulliver.

When the solution has been allowed to settle, the superficial layer of fluid may be drawn off with a pipette, and the deep layer examined for blood corpuscles. These, though quite characteristic if obtained, are rarely to be found in old stains. Occasionally the white corpuscles may be seen when the red have all disappeared. Care must be taken not to confound with blood corpuscles the torula cells which are frequently met with in old blood-stains.

After the microscopical examination, the solution should be submitted to the micro-spectroscope, which as already stated, enables us to determine the presence of the absorption bands and the reducibility of the solution with excessively small quantities. The other chemical tests may then be applied if necessary to small quantities of the coloured solution.

By the above tests, single or combined, blood-stains can, as a rule, be readily identified.

* Bloxam finds that old stains dissolve if heated with water in sealed tubes up to 300° F. (Bowman's "Medical Chemistry," p. 14).

Iron moulds on linen.—These have, as in a case related by Devergie, been mistaken for spots of blood; but the distinction is easy. If the stains are not very old, cold water dissolves the colouring matter of blood more or less completely, but does not affect the iron mould. Hydrochloric acid dissolves out the iron mould, which may be recognised by its appropriate tests; but does not dissolve blood-stains whether recent or old.

Blood-stains on floors, furniture, &c.—Blood that has spouted from an artery on to a wall forms a stain resembling in shape a " point of exclamation" owing to the subsidence of the fluid to the lower end, and its coagulation there. The vertical or the more or less oblique direction of the spot may indicate the position of the wounded vessel. A stain similar to that of an arterial jet may, however, be caused by the splashing of blood on to the walls or furniture.

Blood stains on carpets, &c., may often be detected by bringing a lighted candle to bear on the surface. At the proper angle of incidence the blood-stain may be recognised by its shiny surface, and a scratch with the nail causes on it a vermillion streak. The stains can be examined as if they were stains on linen.

Wood may be shaved off and immersed in water or salt solution, or the stain may be scraped, and the solution made. If the stains are on articles which cannot be immersed, cut, or scraped, a solution may be obtained by placing on the stain moistened filtering paper. This absorbs the colouring matter, and may be used for testing. In applying the guaiacum test to blood colouring matter on filtering paper, it should be borne in mind that some specimens of Swedish filtering paper give of themselves the ozonic reaction.

Blood-stains on articles of steel and iron.—These are readily identified when they present themselves as clots on a clean bright surface of metal. They are then of a clear red! or reddish-brown colour, are easily detached, and scale off under a moderate heat. The presence of animal matter in the spots is readily ascertained by heating them in a reduction-tube, when ammonia is given off, and identified by its alkaline reaction on turmeric paper. A small particle of blood-crust is sufficient for this purpose. The crust placed in a few drops of distilled water will after a time yield a reddish-brown solution and the reactions already described, and if placed under the microscope, will be found to contain blood-globules.

If the blood is smeared on the instrument it will not scale off when heated. The stain must be moistened with distilled water, and carefully scraped off and examined chemically and with the microscope.

If the instrument has been some time exposed to air and moisture, spots of rust will be mixed with those of blood. In this case, too, the stains are not detached by heat, and it will be necessary to scrape them off, place them in distilled water, and separate the insoluble particles of rust by filtration. The resulting coloured liquid will have the chemical and microscopical characters of the blood solution. As, however, the blood colouring matter forms a very insoluble compound with oxide of iron, water may not dissolve it, in which case dilute caustic soda will form a dichroic solution of alkaline hæmatin. Or the mixed blood and rust may be scraped off, heated in a tube with soda or potash, dissolved in water, and treated with the mixed sulphates of iron, and then with hydrochloric acid; Prussian blue will be formed. Rust alone so treated does not give this reaction.

Two other kinds of spots on articles of steel or iron have been pointed out as liable to be mistaken for spots of blood—spots of rust, and spots produced by lemon-juice, vinegar, or other vegetable acid.

Spots of rust.—These somewhat resemble blood-spots in colour, but they do not scale off, and are not soluble in water. If thick enough to be detached, they are readily separated by filtration, leaving the water quite clear, and not affected by the tests for iron. A drop of hydrochloric acid placed on the spot of rust dissolves it, and leaves the metal clean, and on diluting the solution with distilled water, the presence of iron may be detected by appropriate tests.

Spots of lemon-juice.—These have been mistaken for those of blood. A man was suspected of a murder, and a knife, apparently covered with blood, was found in his possession; but on examining it the spots were found to be due to citric acid. The instrument had been used some days before for cutting a lemon, and had been put by unwiped (Orfila).

The thinner spots produced in this way have a reddish-yellow, the thicker a reddish-brown colour, nearly resembling that of blood, and they separate, like blood-spots, when moderately heated. When heated in a tube they give off a volatile matter, which has an acid reaction—spots of blood have an alkaline reaction. The solution in distilled water is light yellow—that of blood is red; it sometimes has an acid reaction—that of blood is neutral, or faintly alkaline; with infusion of galls it yields a black precipitate, a blue with the ferrocyanide, a rich cherry-red with the thiocyanide (sulphocyanide) of potassium. Blood yields a red precipitate with the first test, and is unaffected by the others. The oxide of iron is thrown down by alkalies.

It having been clearly made out that the stain we have been examining is a blood-stain, two questions may arise:

(1) **Is it human blood, or that of an animal ?**

(2) **From what part of the body did it flow ?**

(1) **Is it human blood, or that of an animal ?**—For this two means of diagnosis have been proposed, the one microscopical, the other chemical.

Diagnosis by the microscope.—The only means of distinction under the microscope is afforded by certain well-known differences in the shape and size of the corpuscles. The human blood-corpuscle, depicted in Fig. 52, p. 387, is a circular flattened disc; and that of mammals, with the exception of the camel tribe, has the same form. The only appreciable difference is in the size of the globules. In man they measure on an average $\frac{1}{3200}$ of an inch; in animals the diameters vary from $\frac{1}{3540}$ to $\frac{1}{6300}$ of an inch. But these are only averages; and the extreme measurements, which in man may be stated at $\frac{1}{2000}$ and $\frac{1}{4000}$, lie in some animals still wider apart. When it is borne in mind that in most instances we have to examine a blood solution obtained from dried blood, made to approximate to the average density of blood by the addition of syrup, glycerine, or salt; that the size of the globules is materially affected by the density of the medium in which they float; and that in the blood itself the diameter of one globule may be twice as great as that of another; it is scarcely to be expected that the most skilful and practised person should be able to distinguish human blood from that of other mammals.* But the nucleated

---

* Dr. J. G. Richardson, of Pennsylvania,[1] however, contends that with the use of high powers ($\frac{1}{25}$ to $\frac{1}{50}$ in. objective), and careful micrometic measurements, it is possible, "under favourable conditions," to distinguish positively between the blood corpuscles of man and those of many at least of the domestic animals. Though he admits that it is not possible to distinguish from the human corpuscle that of any animal which measures more than $\frac{1}{4000}$ in., yet he argues that the minimum size of the human corpuscle ($\frac{1}{3021}$ in.) is so much above the average of

---

[1] *Amer. Jour. of Med. Sciences*, July 1874, and various other memoirs.

blood corpuscles of birds, reptiles, and fishes, differ so widely in size and shape from those of man and animals, as to enable us to state positively that the blood in a given case is either that of a mammal, or belongs to one of the three classes of creatures just specified. The differences of size and shape are shown in the annexed wood-cut, in which (1) is human blood, (2) the blood of

FIG. 54.

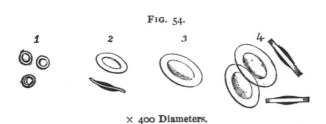

× 400 Diameters.

the common fowl, (3) the blood of the frog, and (4) the blood of a fish. (For some minute details of measurements in Mammalia, see "Micrographic Dictionary," art. Blood, and Plate 39 of that work.)*

Chemical diagnosis.—Barruel first proposed to distinguish the blood of different animals by the characteristic odour given off on adding sulphuric acid. If this acid, diluted with half its bulk of water, is added to the blood of an animal, an odour is perceived which closely resembles that of its perspiration; and probably persons would recognise the odour if informed of its existence, and equally probable that they would be mistaken if asked to name the animal which had supplied the blood.

I make this statement as the result of experiments with the fresh blood of different animals, in such quantity as a drachm or more, made in the class-room for several years in succession. The majority have always been wrong in their guesses; but on one occasion a member of my class was uniformly right in his opinion, though the experiment was so devised as to preclude mere guessing. As a means of distinguishing spots of blood, or solutions obtained

the pig ($\frac{1}{1320}$ in.), the ox ($\frac{1}{1307}$ in.), the red deer ($\frac{1}{1324}$ in.), the cat ($\frac{1}{1404}$ in.), the horse ($\frac{1}{1600}$ in.), the sheep ($\frac{1}{5100}$ in.), the goat ($\frac{1}{6300}$ in.), that the distinction may be made.

* The crystals of hæmoglobin—which may be obtained from *fresh* blood in some animals by mere evaporation, in others with greater difficulty by the aid of ether, freezing, thawing, &c.—differ in different mammals, those of the guinea-pig being tetrahedral, those of the squirrel being hexagonal, the common form being rhombic prisms; but this fact scarcely admits of being applied to medico-legal purposes.

from them, this test must certainly be disallowed. It has utterly failed in the hands of very competent persons (G).

(2) **From what part of the body did it flow?**—It has already been stated that we possess no means of distinguishing menstrual blood from blood from a wound, further than that the nature of the dress, and position of the blood upon it, along with the occurrence of epithelial scales (squamous and cylindrical), may assist us.

In some cases spots submitted for examination are found blended with hair, skin, or mucous membrane, or with other matters adhering to the material on which the blood has fallen. The discovery of such admixtures may often supply very important medico-legal information.

Hair on weapons.—Weapons which have inflicted wounds are generally blood-stained, and we may often discover hairs adhering to the blood-clots, or otherwise attached to the weapon, and it is very important to determine whether the hairs are human hairs or not, and whether they correspond to the hairs on the body of the person who has been wounded; and for this purpose a careful comparison will have to be made of the hairs found on the weapon with those on the body of the deceased. Hairs must not be confounded with fibres of cotton, linen, wool, or silk. Fibres of cotton have a twisted appearance, those of linen have a tapering jointed structure, those of silk are smooth, and those of wool have a peculiar spiral-like imbrication. (Fig. 55.)

Hair consists of a cortical and medullary substance, covered by an imbricated cuticle. When the hair is young and soft, the medullary portion may be absent, and the whole hair has a fibrous appearance. The dark, irregular appearance of the medulla, the striated cortical substance, and the peculiar imbrication of the cuticular scales, render hair easily recognisable. The hairs of the head are usually truncated or split at the free end, while those of the body are, as a rule, pointed, and occasionally this difference may enable us to determine the origin of the hair. The hair of the lower animals differs from human hair in several respects. In many animals the hair is entirely cellular, in others, there is a combination of the cellular with the fibrous structure. Examples of both kinds are given in Fig. 55, which may serve as standards of comparison both as to appearance and size.

FIG. 55.

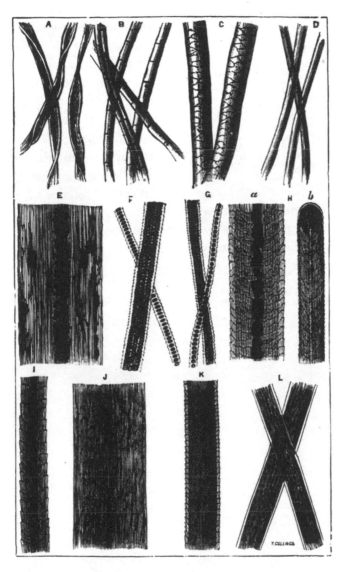

A. Fibres of Cotton. B. of Linen. C. of Wool. D. of Silk.
E. Hair of Pig. F. of Rabbit. G. of Hare. I. of Horse. J. of Cow.
K. of Cat. L. of Dog.
H. Human hair. From head (*a*) ; from body (*b*).

Brain substance on weapons.—Occasionally on weapons which have caused fracture of the skull and laceration of the brain, portions of brain-substance are found. When fresh, it is not easily mistaken; when dry it becomes grey or brown, and horny. When moistened, it assumes a whiter colour and a soapy consistence.

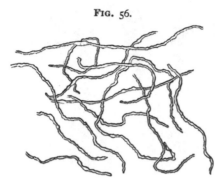

FIG. 56.

Attempts have been made to recognise brain-substance by its reactions with sulphuric and hydrochloric acids; but they are not satisfactory, and may mislead. The only satisfactory method of detection is by the microscope. When the matter is softened in distilled water or in a solution of salt, the presence of nerve cells or of nerve fibres may be ascertained. These are small ($\frac{1}{8000}$ inch or less in diameter), generally ampullated (Fig. 56), or they may have been disorganised, and only myelin drops may remain.

CHAPTER IV.

DEATH BY FIRE—SPONTANEOUS COMBUSTION —DEATH BY LIGHTNING—BY COLD—BY STARVATION.

DEATH BY FIRE.

DEATHS by burns and scalds are of frequent occurrence, and the greater number are due to clothes catching fire, a smaller number to conflagrations, and to explosions of gunpowder, fireworks, and gases. A considerable number of deaths due to scalding liquids are entered in our death registers under "Burns and Scalds," and about fifty deaths in the year are caused by drinking hot water.

The cause of death by burning is not always the same. Some are suffocated by smoke; others die frightened, or by blows from falling bodies; others by the shock that follows extensive injury to the tissues; and others, again, at periods more or less remote from the burning, by collapse, or the effects of inflammation. Children not unfrequently die in a state of coma from severe burns, owing to congestion and serous effusion in the brain, and a frequent cause of death after burns is inflammation of serous or mucous membranes. The duodenum, according to the observations of Curling,* is especially apt to be so affected. The danger from burns and scalds is in great measure proportional to the extent of surface injured.

The appearances produced by burning consist of redness, blisters, entire or burst, roasted patches, sooty spots and marks from burnt articles of clothing, and singed hair.

The same medico-legal questions arise in reference to death by fire as in other forms of external injury, except that the alternative of suicide or homicide rarely presents itself. Both burns and

* "Med. Chir. Trans.," vol. xxv.

scalds are rare suicidal and homicidal acts. In cases of murder, the marks on the body would show that the burning was inflicted during life; but as a murderer sometimes resorts to burning to conceal the real mode and cause of death, we may have to distinguish burning during life from burning after death. Again, when a body is found with marks of burning too extensive to be explained by the quantity of fuel consumed, it may become a question whether it was unusually combustible, or had undergone a process of "spontaneous combustion."

Burns inflicted during life and after death.—The distinction between burns and scalds inflicted before and after death has been made the subject of numerous experiments by Sir R. Christison, Casper, Champouillon, Chambert and others. As a general result of these experiments, it may be stated that the indications of a burn inflicted during life are the presence of vesications and the signs of inflammatory reaction. If these are not present, which may be the case even though the burns have been inflicted during life, we have no means of distinguishing the one from the other. The vesicles, which appear immediately or after a varying interval, contain serum, which either coagulates in mass, or yields a copious precipitate of albumen when heated or acted upon with nitric acid.

Surrounding the vesicle there is a deep red line, which remains after death, and which is a characteristic sign of vital reaction, though it is not always present, as death may occur before it shows itself.

When the cuticle is removed, the skin underneath is found reddened, and dotted by the deep red openings of the sudoriparous and sebaceous ducts. The redness also extends into the subcutaneous tissues. This reddened base of the vesicle is the most valuable indication of a burn inflicted during life, as it will be found where there is no red boundary line. It is scarcely necessary to add that redness follows instantly on the application of heat, and that vesicles show themselves after the interval of a few seconds.

On the other hand, in post-mortem burns vesicles are produced, if at all, with great difficulty. If they do form, they either contain only air, or, if a fluid, one which contains little albumen, and becomes only opaline or milky when heated, or on the addition of nitric acid. The base is not red, but the surface of the skin is of a dull white, dotted with grey at the orifices of the cutaneous ducts. There is no red boundary line. These post-mortem vesicles are most readily produced in anasarcous subjects. Vesicles caused by putrefaction are readily distinguished by the absence of these appearances, the exposed true skin being, like that of adjacent parts, colourless or green.

The appearances just described as due to the application of heat to the living body are common to all intense inflammations of the skin, whether due to disease, or caused by the application of cantharides and other strong irritants, by pressure or by friction. I have seen on the ankles of a young man who had died of acute phthisis, two patches of inflammation of a deep red colour, not removable by pressure, and with well-defined margins, on one of which were large vesicles containing serum. I ascertained beyond doubt that the spots, which had been observed during life, were not caused by the application of any heated body (G.). Appearances simulating burns also precede the acute bed-sore of certain cerebral and spinal affections.*

In all these cases of acute cutaneous inflammation a thin vertical section of the inflamed skin and underlying tissues displays, even to the naked eye, distinct red patches, contrasting very strikingly with similar sections of skin discoloured by mere subsidence of the blood.

The diagnostic marks just described have a distinct bearing on those rare cases in which, as in that of Bolam, tried at Newcastle in 1839, arson is resorted to to conceal the true cause of death.

Of the question of accident, suicide, or homicide, it must suffice to observe that suicides and homicides by fire are very rare ; and that the suicidal cases occur chiefly among persons of unsound mind.

SPONTANEOUS COMBUSTION.

The following case, which rests on the authority of Le Cat, a firm believer in spontaneous combustion, forms a fitting introduction to this subject. It is said to have taken place in 1725 :—

One Millet, of Rheims, was charged with the murder of his wife, the remains of whose body were found lying near the kitchen hearth on the floor, which was partially burnt. Parts of the head and lower extremities, and a few of the vertebræ, had escaped

* Consult Charcot, "Diseases of the Nervous System," Syd. Soc. Trans. 1877.

combustion. Millet stated that he and his wife had retired to rest the previous evening, but that she, not being able to sleep, got up and went into the kitchen, as he supposed, to warm herself; that he was aroused by the smell of fire, and going downstairs, found the deceased lying in the manner stated. The prisoner was condemned to death, but on appeal to a higher court the case was pronounced one of spontaneous human combustion, and the sentence was revoked.

In this case the extent to which the body was consumed gave some support to the opinion that it was unusually combustible, but none to the notion that the fire originated in the body itself. It was certainly in the most favourable circumstances for being *set on fire;* and this is true of most of the cases attributed to spontaneous combustion in England and abroad.

Orfila testifies his belief in spontaneous human combustion by thus describing the phenomena that accompany it :—A light blue flame not readily extinguished by water, but even increased by it, appears over the part about to be attacked, followed by deep eschars, accompanied by convulsions, delirium, vomiting, and diarrhœa. A peculiar state of putrefaction ensues, which soon proves fatal. The process is said to be extremely rapid, but the body is never quite consumed; some parts are only half burnt, while others are reduced to a carbonaceous, fœtid, unctuous ash. The trunk is usually consumed, but the hands and feet escape. The clothes are commonly destroyed; but articles of furniture standing near escape. A thick greasy soot covers the walls and furniture, and the air has an offensive empyreumatic odour. The phenomenon is stated to occur chiefly in aged corpulent females, and especially in persons long addicted to the abuse of spirituous liquors.

It is practically of little consequence whether the doctrine of spontaneous combustion be true or false. The cases* recorded create a presumption in favour of an unusual combustibility of the body, occurring in rare instances, and for the most part in corpu-

* Jacobs, as cited by Casper, has brought together 28, of which 20 occurred in France; and A. Ogston[1] has reported the particulars of a case in which the extent of destruction of the body seemed quite out of proportion to that of the surroundings. A case is also reported in the *Brit. Med. Journal*, 1888 vol. i. p. 841.

[1] *Brit. and For. Med.-Chir. Review*, Jan. 1870.

lent spirit-drinking females, merely requiring to be set on fire, and needing no other fuel but their clothes, night-dress, or ordinary bed-furniture. Till we possess further cases better authenticated and more accurately reported, we must rest content with this amount of knowledge, not forgetting, meanwhile, that such men as Liebig and Casper treat the very notion of spontaneous combustion as an idle fable, stamped with the brand of sheer credulity, and one opposed to such simple facts, among others, as that the human body contains 75 per cent. of water.

The spontaneous combustion of inorganic substances, a subject of much interest and importance, has no medico-legal bearing.

DEATH BY LIGHTNING.

About a score of deaths by lightning occur, one year with another, in England and Wales; of twenty-one deaths, eighteen took place in males and three in females. It is a mode of death that rarely gives rise to medico-legal questions; but as the effects of lightning on the body often resemble those caused by mechanical violence, a question might arise, whether a person found dead under unknown circumstances, had perished by lightning or had been murdered.

Since the introduction of electric lighting several deaths have occurred from an electric shock, owing to workmen inadvertently handling the wires while the current was passing. The cause of death is similar to that of death by lightning; there is, as a rule, no external mark.

In most cases we have a clue to the cause of death in the fact that a thunderstorm has taken place, and that the corpse is found in such a situation, and with such surroundings, as is consistent with its having been struck by lightning.

As a general rule, it may be stated that the electric current prefers good conductors; and as the human body is a very good conductor, it is as likely to be struck as any object similarly situated, unless, perhaps, that object be of metal.

As a general rule, too, lofty objects are most likely to be struck; but persons have been struck in the immediate neighbourhood of tall trees which have been uninjured; and in woods it is not always the highest trees that are struck. The electric discharge is often conducted to the body by such lofty objects as trees, masts, the rigging of ships, and the moist strings of kites. The danger of remaining under a tree during a storm is proverbial.

It has been thought that a person is tolerably safe in an open space far from any object which could attract the electric discharge, but this is an error. The human body may be, in these circumstances, the most prominent object and also the best conductor.

Death may be caused by an electric discharge other than the descending lightning stroke. This happens when a cloud near the earth is negatively electrified, while the earth is positive, and the human body serves as the conductor, by which the equilibrium is restored. This is called the ascending or returning stroke.

The violent mechanical effects produced by the electric discharge —the disruption of buildings and removal of parts of them to a distance, the rending of trees into laths, the separation of good conductors from bad ones, the fusion of metallic substances, the ignition of inflammable ones, the magnetic properties communicated to articles of iron and steel—are familiarly known.

The **post-mortem appearances** in bodies struck by lightning are very various. Sometimes no marks of injury are found, and this is said to occur most commonly in death by the returning stroke. In other cases the body is bruised or torn at the spot where the electric current has entered; or there is merely a small round hole at the point of exit. Extensive bruises and livid streaks are sometimes present, most frequently on the back, and sometimes arborescent markings are visible on the surface of the body (Fig. 57), which are caused by divarications of portions of the discharge, producing a kind of erythema, which indicates the paths followed by the discharge, resembling both in appearance and causation the Lichtenberg figures of experimental electricity. Occasionally, also, metallic chains are fused, causing local burns and metallic streaks on the skin. Fractures of the bones are rare; they may occur, as Ambrose Paré states, without external wound. A case of extensive fracture of the bones of the skull is related by Pouillet. Marks of burns and singeing are sometimes present. They may occur even when the clothes have not been set on fire.

Hunter was of opinion that in death by lightning there was an absence of rigor mortis, that the blood did not coagulate, and that putrefaction was hastened. These statements are not, however, in accordance with other observations in death by lightning; persons killed by lightning being sometimes found rigid in the position in which they were struck. And Richardson's experiments on animals show that well-marked rigidity comes on in death from electrical discharges. The blood seems to coagulate more slowly than usual in these cases, but the course of putrefaction does not seem

FIG. 57.

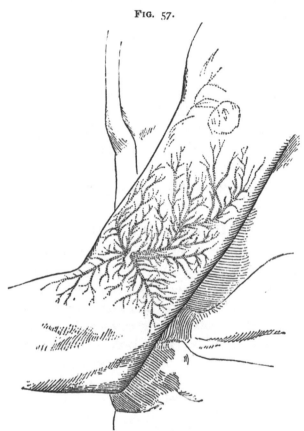

Arborescent markings caused by lightning.
From a Photograph by Mr. Boner of Duns, N.B. (*Lancet*, 1883).

influenced in any appreciable manner. These points are worthy of note; but even should the blood be fluid, rigidity absent, and putrefaction hastened, these are not peculiar to death by lightning, for they may all coincide with other modes of sudden death.

In some cases the state of the objects found on the corpse, or belonging to it, furnish complete evidence of the cause of death. The clothes may be torn and burnt; the shoes struck from the feet; metallic bodies fused and forcibly carried to a distance; and articles of iron or steel, such as the steel of the stays or the main-spring of a watch, rendered strongly magnetic.*

Cause of death.—The electric discharge acts chiefly through the nervous system, and the cause of death is the shock or disruptions sustained by it. When not immediately fatal, its action on the brain, spinal cord, or nerves, is shown by loss of sight, and various affections of sensation or voluntary motion, temporary or permanent.

It has been recommended that executions should take place by electricity, and in August 1890, at Auburn, in the United States, a murderer, Kemmler, was so executed, the current being introduced into the body at the shaven scalp. At the post-mortem examination, there was a well-defined mark on the scalp where the skin had been scorched, and a similar spot on the small of the back, where the second electrode was placed, below these the blood was found to be converted into a carbonaceous mass. The body was much burned and soon become rigid ; the organs were generally healthy.†

DEATH BY COLD.

This is an uncommon event in this country, though death by cold and inanition combined is not very rare in severe winters.

The first effect of intense cold is a sense of numbness and stiffness in the muscles of the limbs and face. This is soon followed by torpor and profound sleep, passing into coma and death.

The effect of cold on the circulation is to drive the blood from the surface to the interior of the body, so as to gorge the spleen, liver, lungs, and brain. The genital organs are also congested, sometimes giving rise to priapism. The temperature of the blood itself is lowered ; the heart contracts slowly and feebly, and the pulse is small and weak. The congestion of the nervous centres occasions numbness, torpor, somnolency, giddiness, dimness of sight, tetanus, and paralysis ; and the congestion of the brain sometimes occasions a species of delirium, as happened to Edward Jenner ; or the appearance of intoxication, as witnessed by Captain Parry and others in the expeditions to the North Pole.

---

* A full description of the effects of lightning will be found in Dr. Sistier's work, " De la Foudre," Paris, 1766. See also an interesting series of experiments on animals with powerful electric discharges, by Sir B. W. Richardson, *Med. Times and Gaz.*, May, August and September 1869.

† *Brit. Med. Journ.*, 1890, vol. ii. p. 354.

The effect of cold varies in intensity with sex, age, and strength : the very young, the aged, the infirm, persons worn out by disease and fatigue, and those addicted to the use of intoxicating liquors, perish soonest. Some persons, too, have a great advantage over others in their power of resisting cold—a fact frequently observed by voyagers and travellers in the Arctic regions.

In estimating the effect of cold, it should be borne in mind that the body is cooled in three ways—by evaporation, by conduction of the air in contact with it, and by radiation.

The cutaneous evaporation is increased by dry and diminished by moist air. Hence the body parts with its heat more rapidly in a dry atmosphere. On the other hand, the body is cooled by conduction when the air is moist ; so that the body is cooled alike by dry cold air and by cold moist air. Cold humid winds lower the temperature in a very striking degree by evaporation and by conduction. The effect of a slight breeze in increasing the sensation of cold has been remarkably shown in the expeditions to the Polar seas.

Post-mortem appearances.—The appearances after death by cold still require investigation, but the following have been found by Ogston* uniformly present in adults : A florid or arterial hue of the blood, except when in mass; an over-distension of both cavities of the heart and all the large vascular trunks ; a notable pallor of the skin generally, but here and there dusky red patches on non-dependent parts. He found also, as a rule, anæmia of the viscera most largely supplied with blood. In ten cases he found moderate congestion of the brain in three, and of the liver in seven. Other observers have, however, described the viscera as being congested. In two cases reported by Dr. Kellie, of Leith, there was a large effusion of serum in the ventricles of the brain. Though the appearances described by Ogston seem to be the most reliable and uniform, further investigations will be necessary before we can consider them as altogether characteristic and conclusive of death from cold.

The question of accident, suicide, or homicide rarely finds place in this mode of death ; but in one singular and horrible case death by cold was a homicidal act. A girl, 11 years of age, some years since, was compelled by her parents to stand naked in a pail of ice-cold water, while the water was being poured over her, till she died.

* "Lect. on Med. Jurisp.," p. 556.

DEATH BY STARVATION.

This is a very rare event; but death from cold in persons in-sufficiently nourished is not infrequent. Cases of homicide by the deprivation of food are of occasional occurrence;* the insane sometimes commit suicide by obstinately refusing to take suste-nance; some prisoners under long sentences would starve them-selves if not fed by force.

The symptoms produced by protracted abstinence are pain in the epigastrium, relieved by pressure, with intense thirst and extreme weakness and emaciation. The face is pale and ghastly; the cheeks are sunken; the eyes hollow, wild, and glistening; the breath hot; the mouth dry and parched; the bones project. The body at length exhales a fœtid odour, the mucous membranes of the outlets become red and inflamed, and death takes place in a fit of maniacal delirium, or in horrible convulsions.

From Willan's case, presently to be cited, and the statements of prisoners who have voluntarily abstained, it appears that the craving for food disappears in about three days, and that the second day of abstinence is that of greatest suffering (G.).

Post-mortem appearances.—The body is much emaciated, and exhales a fœtid odour; the eyes are red and open; the skin, mouth, and fauces dry; the stomach and intestines empty and contracted, so as to be quite translucent; the gall-bladder is distended with bile; the heart, lungs, and large vessels are col-lapsed, bloodless and attenuated; and putrefaction runs a rapid course. These appearances are not so characteristic as to be decisive of the mode of death; but in the absence of any disease productive of extreme emaciation such a state of body furnishes a strong presumption of death by starvation. It must be recollected that there are maladies, such as stricture of the œsophagus and organic disease of the stomach, tubercular disease, diabetes, Addison's disease, &c., which prove fatal by starvation or mal-nutrition. Search should therefore be made for such causes of death.

* The Penge case (Central Criminal Court, Sept. 1877) involved a charge of homicide by starvation against four persons. The prisoners were convicted of murder, but owing to objections urged against the valadity of the medical evidence for the prosecution, the sentence was commuted. For an account of the post-mortem appearances, and discussion of their significance, see the *Brit. Med. Journ.*, Oct. 6, 1877, *et seq.*

The post-mortem appearances were faithfully described by Mr. Biggs in the case of Mark Cornish, killed by starvation and exposure by his father and stepmother.* He stated at the inquest that the deceased was so wasted that he had scarcely any muscle left, and no fat; that he looked like a skeleton with the skin tightly stretched over him; that he could not only see each bone, but its peculiarities; that all the organs were healthy, though the heart and stomach were small; that the omentum was as clear as glass; that there was no food in the stomach; that the small intestines were nearly empty; and that there was no appearance of chyle.

The period at which death happens varies with age, sex, strength, and amount of exertion, and especially with the supply of water.

The question, how long a person may remain without food, or with a very scanty supply of it, is of some importance, as will appear from the case of Elizabeth Canning, quoted in Dr. Cumming's Lectures.† It was alleged that a girl of 18 had been confined, in the depth of winter, twenty-eight days, without fire, with about a gallon of water in a pitcher, and with no food but some pieces of bread, amounting altogether to about a quartern loaf, and a small mince-pie which she happened to have in her pocket, and that at the expiration of the period she retained strength enough to break down a window-shutter fastened with nails, get out of the window on to a sort of pent-house, thence jump to the ground nine or ten feet, and finish by walking from Enfield Wash to Aldermanbury.

The cases presently to be cited give good ground for believing that life might have been prolonged for twenty-eight days, even more, on this scanty supply of nourishment; but it is extremely improbable that at the end of this time Elizabeth Canning could have had strength enough left to effect her escape. This case is also curious in its bearing on the question of identity. A fresh interest has been given to this question of prolonged abstinence by the case of Sarah Jacob, the Welsh Fasting Girl.

There are four distinct classes of cases which may be used to throw light on this question of the duration of life under complete, or nearly complete, deprivation of food: 1. Mechanical obstruction of the gullet; 2. Shipwrecked persons subject to exposure and

---

* *Morning Chronicle*, February 26, 1853.
† *Medical Gazette*, vol. xix.

fatigue; 3. Persons buried, and rendered inactive, by such obstructions as falling earth; 4. Persons wilfully abstaining from food, generally under circumstances demanding little exertion of mind or body.

1. For an interesting case of this class we are indebted to Dr. Currie, of Liverpool. A man, 66 years of age, survived a complete obstruction of the gullet (with the aid of nutritious clysters and baths of milk-and-water administered during thirty-two days) for thirty-six days. The man, who was tall and corpulent, was reduced from an ascertained weight of 240 lbs. down to 138 lbs.—a loss of 102 lbs., of which two-fifths took place in the space of thirty-two days, for his weight before the complete obstruction of the gullet was 179 lbs. In the last twelve days he lost 16 lbs., or at the rate of $1\frac{3}{4}$ lb. per diem; and this loss the already wasted frame sustained in spite of the nourishment administered in the mode just described. What the unchecked rate of waste would have been we have no means of ascertaining; but we know that death took place when the body had lost 102 lbs. out of 240, or little more than two parts in five of its original weight—a reduction corresponding most closely to the results of Chossat's experiments on animals. He laid it down as a broad principle, derived from experiments on many different living creatures, that life ceases when an animal loses two-fifths of its weight; so that an animal weighing 100 lbs. would die when its weight was reduced to 60 lbs. Though life may cease before this point is attained, and the period varies greatly in different classes of animals, it can rarely extend beyond it. The daily loss amounts to one twenty-fourth of the entire weight —a statement in harmony with the conclusion of Bidder and Schmidt, that an animal, to maintain its weight, ought to take one twenty-third part of it daily in the shape of food susceptible of being assimilated, water, oxygen, and inorganic salts of course included.

The progressive and rapid waste of the body, and the extinction of life at or about the point at which an animal loses two-fifths of its weight, may therefore be taken as data sufficiently established; as also the fact, long since proved by Redi, that animals live much longer (birds more than twice as long) when they have free access to water.

2. Of the prolongation of life under the fatigue, exposure, total privation of food, and want of fresh water (except such as may

have been supplied by dew or rain) incidental to shipwrecks, we have some well-authenticated cases. A narrative of a shipwreck on the Calcutta coast, which has been placed at my disposal, shows that out of eighteen men without food or water twelve days, three died, the rest escaped and recovered (G.). And a very detailed and evidently faithful account of the picking up at sea of Captain Casey, commander of the *Jane Lowden*, timber vessel, shows that out of eighteen men, including the captain himself, wholly without provisions and fresh water, one survived eleven days, one twelve, one fourteen, two fifteen, one eighteen, and the captain himself, who recovered, twenty-eight days. Two men appear to have died early, furiously delirious; one (a lad, aged 19) who died on the twelfth day, was quietly delirious, with spectral illusions; two others were delirious, and Captain Casey had illusions of hearing. *

3. Of confinement in coal mines we have instances of men and boys surviving six and eight days, and one man twenty-three days.† There was access to water for the first ten days.

4. The longest abstinence from food, with free access to water, of which I have had experience among prisoners, is ten days. In two men and one woman complete abstinence from food during this period was followed by no bad symptom, and the ordinary prison diet was resumed without injury to health. The prisoners were weakened, but by no means exhausted (G.). In the case of ten days' starvation of a prisoner reported by Casper, scarcely any liquid was taken, and the exhaustion was much greater.‡

The case of Bernard Cavanagh, though not one of complete abstinence, may be added to the foregoing. Having been committed to gaol for three months, he was placed in a cell under strict surveillance, and refused to eat or drink. This continued, as it was alleged, nine days, at the end of which time he was reported to be in "perfect bodily health." But on the thirteenth day it was remarked that the gruel supplied to him came back the same in quantity, but much thinner. The man's health having by this time suffered, he was supplied with, and gladly received, nourishing food.§

But we have well authenticated cases extending much beyond

* The *Times*, February 7, 1866.
† Dr. Sloan, *Med. Gaz.*, vol. xvii. pp. 264 and 389.
‡ "Handbook," vol. ii. p. 28. § *Medical Times*, December 4, 1841.

ten days. There is Hufeland's curious case of the ruined merchant, a suicide by starvation, who kept a diary of his sensations for thirteen days, and died on the 18th (G. H. Lewes' "Physiology of Common Life," vol. i. p. 25); the case of Viterbi, who survived twenty-one days; of Cecilia Rygeway, reported to have survived forty-days; and a case of forty-two days, briefly attested by Van Swieten. The third of these cases is thus epitomised by the author of an article on Fasting Girls published in *All the Year Round*, Oct. 9, 1869: "Cecilia de Rygeway, having been imprisoned in Nottingham jail for the murder of her husband during the reign of Edward III. (the year 1357), remained 'mute and abstinent' for forty days, neither eating nor drinking during this time. It was considered so much in the nature of a religious sign or miracle that Dame Rygeway was pardoned by the king." The fourth case is briefly mentioned by Van Swieten in his "Commentaries on Boerhaave's Aphorisms" (heading, Melancholy Madness): "I knew a woman," he says, "who obstinately refused all kinds of nourishment for six weeks, drinking nothing but a little water at intervals, so that at length she perished, quite juiceless and dried up."

From March to May 1890* an Italian named Succi underwent a voluntary fast of forty days, apparently with no ill effect; he had, however, free access to simple liquids and occasionally took a narcotic; after the fast he gradually reverted to a solid dietary.

Alexandre Jacques† fasted for fifty days, taking only mineral water and a limited quantity of a secret powder obtained, he said, from herbs at Crayford. His loss of weight was not regular; he passed about 20 ozs. of urine daily, but some days he voided none at all; the bowels were evacuated on the thirty-seventh day by enemata. He suffered during the latter part of the fast from gout; as a rule he slept well; the excretion of urea diminished to a minimum of 114 grs. per diem, the average being 144 grs.; he smoked cigarettes continually during the fifty days, some 700 in number.

Willan's well-authenticated and minutely-detailed case of voluntary starvation‡ occurred in the person of a young man, a religious

* *Brit. Med. Journ.*, 1890, vol. i. p. 1444.

† *Ibid.*, 1891, vol. ii. p. 710.

‡ Miscellaneous Works of the late Robert Willan, M.D., F.R.S., &c., edited by Ashby Smith, M.D., 1821 (p. 437). Willan, in commenting on this case, cites the following cases:—

1. "Mémoires de l'Académie des Sciences," 1769. A madman lived forty-seven

maniac, who drank water and a little orange-juice, but ate nothing, and lived sixty-one days, and then, being cautiously fed, other eighteen days. This survivorship of sixty-one days without food gives an air of probability to the French case of Guillaume Granét, the prisoner of Toulouse, which was reported to the Academy of Medicine as follows: He resorted to starvation to avoid punishment. For the first seven days the symptoms were not very remarkable; his face was flushed, his breath foul, and his pulse small and feeble. After this period he was compelled to drink water occasionally, to relieve his excessive thirst, but in spite of the close watch kept over him, he frequently drank his urine, or the water of the prison kennel. His strength did not appear to fail him during the greater part of the time, and, with varying symptoms of constitutional disturbance and acute sufferings, he lingered to the fifty-eighth day, when he expired, after struggling four hours in convulsions.*

From the best authenticated cases of prolonged abstinence, whether voluntary or involuntary, we infer that, though life may be prolonged up to the limit of about two months, there is progressive and rapid loss of weight, and at length extreme emaciation. If, then, it were alleged by or on behalf of some man, woman, or child, that there had been a total abstinence from food for some period exceeding two months, or abstinence, not from food only, but from water also, for some such period as one month, we should be justified in looking on the case with the utmost possible suspicion, especially if the person so abstaining, having anything approaching the plumpness and fresh colour belonging to health, were to assert that no action of the bowels or bladder had taken place. The making such person the subject of exhibition, and, still worse, of gain, would add indignation to doubt, and leave no alternative but to demand the decisive test of the closest surveillance.

Two English cases, in which this severe test was applied, are on record: the one the fasting woman of Tutbury, the other the

days with nothing but a pint and a half of water per day. He stood constantly in the same position for thirty-eight days of that time, but during the remaining eight lay down, and then took nothing, not even water. When he first began to eat again, he recovered his reason, but soon relapsed. 2. "Edin. Med. Essays," vol. vi. A young girl fasted, at one time thirty-four, at another fifty-four days, from a spasm or some obstruction of the œsophagus.

* Foderé, vol. ii. p. 276.

fasting girl of Wales; for we pass over all cases not thus tested. Ann Moore, the fasting woman of Tutbury, was 58 years old in 1808, when she asserted that she had gone twenty months without food. She said that four years before that date she had a severe illness, which lasted thirteen weeks, followed by incomplete recovery, for she was subject for months afterwards to violent fits and spasms at frequent and irregular intervals. A year later she had another severe illness that lasted eleven weeks, and was followed by loss of appetite and indigestion, increased in 1806 by nursing a boy affected with a repulsive disease. From October in that year to February 1807 she ate a penny loaf in a fortnight, and drank a little tea without milk or sugar. From that time till November 1808 she lived, she said, only on water and tea. The case having been published in the *Monthly Magazine* early in 1809, created a great sensation, and led to donations of money, on which the woman lived four years. But in 1813 a few scientific men in the neighbourhood determined to sift the matter to the bottom. They got her to consent to have her room guarded and watched. This was done during nine days, at the end of which time she gave in, being terribly emaciated, and now really almost starved to death. She asked for food, recovered her strength, and set her mark to a written confession, in which she admitted that she had occasionally taken nourishment during the last six years, and humbly asked pardon of God and man for the wicked deception she had practised.*

Sarah Jacob, daughter of Evan Jacob, a respectable and solvent tenant farmer, was the third child of a healthy family of seven, living in a mean-looking house, with thatched roof and clay floor, in which the girl and her parents occupied the same small bedroom, She was born May 12, 1857; her case began to attract public attention in 1867, when she was more than 10 years old; and she died December 7, 1869, a little more than 12½ years of age. She was a fair, good-looking child, intelligent and precocious, impressionable and emotional, fond of finery, and addicted to the reading

---

* This history of Ann Moore is a further abbreviation of the abstract given in *All the Year Round.* The account of the Welsh Fasting Girl is taken from Dr. Fowler's work, which derives a special interest from the prominent part played by its author in the case from first to last—"A Complete History of the Case of the Welsh Fasting Girl (Sarah Jacob), with Comments thereon ; and Observations on Death from Starvation," by Robert Fowler, M.D. Edin., &c. 1871.

of religious books and the reciting and composing of verses. In February 1866, when nearly nine years old, she had an attack of scarlet fever, followed by acute pain of stomach and vomiting of blood; and from this time she was alleged to have kept her bed. The pain and vomiting were soon followed by strong convulsions, with arching backward of the body, and symptoms of pleurisy. The body remained rigid for a month; she took little food, and grew thin. In April 1867 she was treated for inflammation of the brain, and about this time is stated to have taken no food for a month, though the lips were moistened from time to time with beer, and only scanty evacuations of either kind were passed. After the inflammatory attack she lost her hair. The fits, which had been convulsive, now changed to short losses of consciousness, with sudden wakings and throwing about of the arms; and the left leg was stated to be rigid. On the 10th of October of this year (1867) she is said to have ceased to take any kind of food; on the 6th of the following month to have had the last discharge from the bowels; and at the end of it to have passed urine for the last time.

We glean from the detailed accounts of the case that the father asserted, and the public were asked to believe, that this girl took no food whatever for two years and two months, and the last week of watching; and nevertheless, during the first three weeks of this total abstinence the bowels were not only frequently and largely relieved (possibly of matters collected previously), but that the usual quantity of water was passed for several weeks; that the hair which had fallen off, grew again, thick and long; that her naturally healthy look was more than maintained, and her bulk apparently increased.

It was at the period to which we are referring (October 1867) that visits of curiosity commenced, and soon became common, followed by their natural consequences—presents of money and books, mostly religious. The girl was gaily and fantastically dressed, and got up for show, somewhat after the fashion of a bride. By the end of the year 1868 the case became so notorious that visits grew more and more numerous, railways and local guides coming into requisition. A local reporter and several medical visitors now appear on the stage. In the spring of 1869 a public meeting was held, and a watching committee appointed, whose inefficiency and failure are duly reported at p. 22 of Dr. Fowler's work. Other visits of inquiring and intelligent persons followed, and on the 7th of September 1869, Dr. Fowler wrote a letter to the *Times* giving the results of a careful and judicious inquiry, carried as far as the parents would permit, and giving it as his opinion that Sarah Jacob was deceiving her parents, and that it was not possible to state what part of the symptoms resulted from "a morbid perversion of will," and what from "intentional deceit."

The complete publicity thus given to the case led, by steps not necessary to describe, to the selection of four trained nurses from Guy's Hospital, to visit and keep constant watch over Sarah Jacob, in order to ascertain whether she got food and drink, or not. Certain medical men were also selected as visitors. An early result of this procedure was to disprove one of the assertions made by the parents, to the effect that the usual discharges from the bowels and bladder were absent. The history of the case from day to day is one of gradual loss of strength, development of feverishness, restlessness, and occasional delirium, progressive quickening of the pulse, and the exhalation from the body and breath of a very peculiar and highly offensive odour. In spite of the warnings given to the father, no food or drink was supplied, and on the eighth day the girl died, exhausted and insensible.

On the 21st of December 1869 an inquest was held, and evidence given as to the state of the body after death. It was plump and well formed, and covered with fat from half an inch to an inch thick; there was no obstruction in any part of the alimentary canal, and all the important organs of the body were sound. The body was perfectly free from disease. The jury brought in a verdict to the effect that Sarah Jacob died from starvation caused by the father's neglecting to induce her to take food. The father was accordingly committed for manslaughter, but admitted to bail. The case was then taken up by the Government, and on the 26th of February 1870 summonses were served on the five medical men who had been in attendance during the watching, and on the parents of the girl; and a ten days' inquiry was held before the bench of magistrates, adjourned, and resumed. The result of the inquiry was the acquittal of the medical men, but the committal for trial at the next assizes of the parents, Evan and Hannah Jacob. On the 13th of July 1870 the grand jury found a true bill, and the following day the trial took place, which issued in a verdict of guilty against both parents, with a recommendation to mercy of the mother.

Sarah Jacob evidently succumbed to the form of starvation that proved fatal to the three who died among the thirteen shipwrecked sailors whose cases are given above, and to those who perished soonest among the eighteen, of whom Captain Casey was the solitary survivor on the 28th day. In these instances death took place, under privation and exposure, in less than twelve days; and we have now to add the death on the eighth day of a girl twelve and a half years old, apparently healthy, but ill-prepared for total abstinence from food and drink by more than two years spent chiefly in bed, dating from a recovery, not complete, from a series of maladies, comprising scarlet fever, acute gastric derangement, symptoms attributed to inflammation of the brain, pleurisy, and anomalous rigid spasms of some continuance.

To these quicker deaths, attended only by slight loss of substance, the analogy of medical nomenclature justifies us in applying the term acute starvation. If this term be accepted as descriptive of these cases, and the limit of survivorship be taken at two weeks, we shall be justified in characterising as chronic starvation those in which the abstinence from food (complete, or nearly so) has extended to the extreme limit of two months. In the first class the body may be found well nourished; in the last reduced to the extreme described by Dr. Willan as "emaciated to a most astonishing degree," or, in the words of Mr. Biggs, "like a skeleton with the skin tightly stretched over him:" so that "he could not only see each bone, but its peculiarities."

An interesting case bearing on this subject is that of Reg. v. Justan, 4 Feb. 1893, Crown Cases Reserved, in which the prisoner lived alone with her sick and helpless aunt and neglected to give to her aunt such assistance as was necessary in order to enable her to obtain food and medical attendance, and neglected also to inform persons, able and willing to give assistance, of her aunt's condition. It being found as a fact that her negligence accelerated her aunt's death, it was held she was properly convicted of manslaughter.

The moral obligation to assist a sick and helpless person imposes a legal duty not to withhold such assistance, and, consequently, a person who wilfully neglects to enable a sick person to obtain such food and medicine as may be necessary to sustain life is guilty of manslaughter.

PART III.

—•••—

TOXICOLOGY.

THE frequent occurrence of cases of real or supposed poisoning, and the complicated nature of the questions to which they give rise, render this not only the most interesting, but the most important division of Forensic Medicine; while the great number of recognised poisonous agents causes it to occupy no inconsiderable part of every medico-legal treatise.

Before proceeding to treat of the Poisons in detail, certain questions relating to poisons and poisoning in general will have to be discussed, such as the definition of the word poison, the mode of action of poisons, the causes which modify their action, and the classification of which they are susceptible.

It will also be necessary to point out the means we possess of answering the many questions which present themselves for solution when a suspicion of poisoning has been raised, and we are required to determine whether it is well or ill-founded. Under this head we shall have to discuss the inferences that may be drawn from the origin and progress of the symptoms which gave rise to the suspicion; the value and significance of post-mortem appearances when death happens; and the light that may be thrown upon the case by experiments on animals, by chemical analysis, and by the conduct of suspected persons.

Again, the precautions which ought to be observed in conducting post-mortem examinations in cases of suspected poisoning, and those, equally important, which should be borne in mind in the several steps of a chemical investigation, ought to be very carefully examined and explained.

These leading divisions of the subject of poisoning will be treated with some detail in three separate chapters, being so many departments of the principal subject of POISONS IN GENERAL.

CHAPTER I.

DEFINITION OF A POISON—ACTION AND CLASSIFICATION OF POISONS.

1. **Definition of a Poison.** — The meaning which ought to attach to the word poison is best ascertained by a simple process of exclusion. A substance that affects one person through peculiarity of constitution, but has no effect on others, is not a poison: a substance which owes its effect to some temporary condition of system, as when cold water is swallowed by a person heated by exercise, is not a poison; substances which mechanically injure and inflame the internal parts, such as pins and needles, and particles of steel or glass, are not poisons; again, hot water, the water being merely a vehicle for heat, is not a poison. Substances, therefore, which owe their action to some peculiarity of constitution, or unusual condition of the body; mechanical irritants, and harmless substances rendered injurious by extraneous causes, are not properly termed poisons. Nor does the mode of application form any part of the definition of the word. Whether applied to the skin, or inhaled, or swallowed, or introduced into the anus or vagina, ear or nostril, it is still a poison. Again, the quantity that may prove fatal, or the time required to destroy life, cannot enter into the definition; nor can the form of the substance or matter, whether solid, liquid, or gaseous, be held to be material. These exclusions have narrowed the possible definition of a poison, so that the following may be accepted as sufficient for every practical purpose:—**A poison is any substance or matter (solid, liquid, or gaseous) which, when applied to the body outwardly, or in any way introduced into it, can destroy life by its own inherent qualities, without acting mechanically, and irrespective of temperature.**

In the great majority of cases poisons are swallowed. They are " given to," administered to," or " taken by " the person injured or killed; but they have been introduced into the body through the lungs, rectum, vagina, ear, or nostril. They have also been applied by subcutaneous injection, or to the skin unbroken or abraded.

The word "poison" is often qualified by such terms as "active," "virulent," "deadly"; and the last of these terms is very generally used in indictments.

A "deadly" poison may mean one that is fatal in a small dose, or kills quickly in a larger one, or which, irrespective of the dose, is more dangerous or difficult to counteract than others. Strychnine and oxalic acid, for instance, are both "deadly poisons"; but while less than a grain of the one and less than half an ounce of the other may destroy life, a full dose of oxalic acid may kill much more quickly than even a large dose of strychnine. On the other hand, the fatal dose of Epsom salts or sulphate of potassium is two or three ounces, and even those quantities would not prove certainly or rapidly fatal; so that it would be incorrect to call these substances "deadly poisons." Nor would the term be rightly applied to such a substance as sulphate of zinc, which is often prescribed as an emetic in doses of a scruple or half a drachm; or to the non-corrosive preparations of mercury, iron, or copper. In any case the term "deadly poison" is open to the objection of raising an unnecessary verbal question; and when used in indictments should be treated as mere "legal surplusage," in accordance with the wise dictum of Mr. Justice Erle.

"A destructive thing," a phrase also used in indictments, if not a poison properly so called, must be some substance or matter which kills by a mechanical action on the internal parts, or by some adventitious property, such as heat. Particles of glass or steel, by irritating the lining membrane of the alimentary canal; pins and needles, by wounding vital organs, or inflaming less important parts; and hot water, by causing fatal inflammation, may be regarded as "destructive things"; but it is doubtful whether the term would apply to such matters as sponge or plaster of Paris, which may destroy life by blocking the passage of the intestines.*

* It would appear from a decision (Court for Crown Cases Reserved— Queen v. Cramp, Times, March 1, 1880), that the element of quantity must be taken into consideration in the legal definition of a "noxious thing." The prisoner was indicted for having administered a "noxious thing"—half an ounce of oil of juniper, with intent to cause abortion. He was convicted; but an appeal was lodged on the ground that the thing must be noxious in itself,

Having defined the term "poison" with sufficient precision to indicate the matters which will have to be examined in the following pages, certain general questions relating to poisons must next be considered. These are—Their **mode of action,** and the **causes which modify their action.**

2. **Mode of action of poisons.**—This is twofold, **local,** and **remote.**

Their **local action** may consist in **corrosion,** or chemical decomposition, as when a strong acid, a caustic alkali, or a corrosive salt, is applied externally or taken internally: in **inflammation,** followed by adhesion, suppuration, ulceration, or gangrene, when such irritants as arsenic, tartar-emetic, or cantharides are similarly taken or applied; and lastly, in an **effect on the nerves** of sensation or motion. The numbness and tingling of the lips, tongue, and throat, occasioned by chewing monkshood (or the local application of cocaine), the sharp, pricking sensation in the tongue caused by the Arum maculatum, and the numbness of the skin which ensues on the application of prussic acid, chloroform, or veratrine, are instances of local action on the nerves of sensation; while the palsy, due to the direct application of opium, ticunas, or prussic acid to the muscles, the dilatation of the pupil from the application of belladonna, and its contraction under the use of the Calabar bean, illustrate the same local action on motion.

Remote action is of two kinds, **reflex** and **specific.** The **reflex** effects start from the point of local action of the poison, as in the effect on the heart produced by the corrosive acid poisons. The specific effects are the result of the special action of the poison on particular organs or parts of the body, as may be noted in the symptoms caused by such a poison as arsenic, which when swallowed, and so applied to the lining membrane of the alimentary canal, gives rise to the same cramps as cholera, English and Asiatic; but the same poison inserted into a wound, applied to the skin, or inhaled, inflames the mucous surfaces with which it

and not merely when administered in excess. Lord Coleridge, in pronouncing judgment, held that there was no substance deemed poisonous which might not be salutary in certain medicinal doses; that the reasonable construction in every case is a question for the jury, whether the substance under the circumstances of its administration is a noxious thing or not. "If a person administers, with intent to procure miscarriage, something which, as administered, is 'noxious,' he administers a 'noxious thing.'"

does not come into immediate contact. This is its specific action. Again, oxalic acid, which acts on the stomach as a corrosive and violent irritant, causes the same constitutional shock which attends all severe local injuries. This is its remote reflex effect; but it has also a remote specific effect on the heart and nervous system. The purest example of a remote reflex effect of a common kind is afforded by the mineral acids, and the alkalies and their carbonates, which, by the local destruction they occasion, give rise to the symptoms of collapse present in extensive burns and scalds. This absence of remote specific effects has led some authors to doubt the propriety of classing these chemicals among poisons.

A knowledge of the **specific** remote action of poisons is of the first importance, for it often enables us to define the class to which a poison belongs, and even to indicate the very poison itself. Individual poisons select different organs or systems of the body, on which they exert their special or specific action. Thus, on the brain, some poisons, such as those of the narcotic class, act as depressants, producing stupor; others act as excitants, such as the belladonna group, producing delirium; on the spinal cord, some cause paralysis, such as tobacco, aconite, and Calabar bean; others, again, excite the nerve cells, producing tetanic spasms, such as strychnine; while curare and hemlock are examples of poisons acting on the motor-nerve endings, producing paralysis. Arsenic sets up inflammation in the mucous membranes, mercury attacks the salivary glands and mouth, cantharides the urinary system, chromate of potassium the conjunctiva, iodine the lymphatic glands, phosphorus affects the liver, and spurred rye produces gangrene of the limbs. Poisonous substances used in the arts also reveal themselves through their specific actions. Thus the dropped hand betrays the use of lead, a tremor like paralysis agitans that of mercury, gangrene of the jaws that of phosphorus, and a peculiar rash about the nostrils, ears, bends of the arms, and scrotum that of the arsenite of copper.

These statements might lead to serious mistakes if it were not understood that some constant symptoms of these poisons are also occasional symptoms of others. Thus, tetanic spasms, so characteristic of the action of strychnine, may occur in poisoning by morphine and other of the alkaloids, as well as by arsenic, corrosive sublimate, and tartar-emetic. Salivation, again, may result from poisons other than mercury; and the dropped hand from the preparations of arsenic as well as from lead. Nor should it be forgotten that these are but the leading phenomena among a considerable group of less characteristic symptoms. Thus, severe irritation of the alimentary canal, inflammation of all the mucous surfaces, a rapid pulse, a series of acute nervous symptoms, and a cutaneous rush, may all occur in a case of arsenical poisoning; and the same is true of oxalic acid and the salts of mercury. It must also be understood that many of the best-marked symptoms of poisoning are also symptoms of disease—a fact that will be fully illustrated in the chapter which treats of the Evidence of Poisoning (p. 428).

Some poisons produce their fatal results by a reflex effect on the heart and general system, such as the strong mineral acids; but to produce their remote specific effects, poisons must be absorbed and carried with the blood to the parts affected. That poisons are absorbed and circulated through the system, in whatever way the poison is applied or introduced, is proved by the analysis of the blood, secretions, and solid textures; and the list of poisons thus detected includes every substance which can be recognised by its odour or colour, or which (not having been completely decomposed) can be submitted to chemical reagents.

The majority of poisons produce their fatal results by their specific effects on the organs to which they are carried by the blood-stream, or in some cases by the lymphatics. Claude Bernard conclusively showed this by experiments demonstrating the specific and selective action of curara on motor nerves; while Magendie had previously shown that the spasms caused by strychnine were due to an action on the spinal cord. Many other examples might be cited showing this specific or selective action of poisons: thus, besides those just mentioned, some poisons paralyse the heart, others the respiration, while still others attack the brain.

The rapidity of the action of a poison is as a rule in direct proportion to the rapidity of its absorption. Thus, speaking generally, poisons act more quickly when introduced into a vein or under the skin than when taken into the stomach. In the last instance, excretion may be so rapid that poisoning does not occur at all—as, e.g., a dose of curara may be administered without effect by the stomach to an animal, which, given subcutaneously, would produce death; but if, after it has reached the stomach, the renal arteries be tied so as to stop excretion, the animal dies with signs of curara poisoning.

The theory of absorption finds a practical application in the use of ligatures, cupping-glasses, and lip-suction, in the case of poisons inserted into wounds.

Besides their specific action, some poisons seem to kill any protoplasm with which they come into contact: such are called "protoplasmic" poisons.

Poisons also act by diffusion, as when, *e.g.*, extensive inflammation, suppuration, and sloughing follow the bite of a rattlesnake. An analogous example may be instanced in acute spreading gangrene.

3. **The causes which modify the action of poisons** are three in number :—**Their quantity and form. The part to which they are applied. The condition of the body itself.**

Quantity and form.—Quantity.—As a general rule, the larger the quantity of a poison the more prompt and severe its action; but a large dose of a poison that is swallowed may be immediately and completely discharged, while a smaller dose may be retained and prove fatal. The action of some poisons also varies remarkably in kind as well as degree with the quantity taken. Thus, a large dose of oxalic acid may kill almost instantly by shock; a smaller dose may still prove fatal by acting on the heart; a yet smaller dose affects chiefly the spinal cord; and a more minute dose still, the brain. Again, small repeated doses will develop other symptoms than a single large dose. Of the whole class of narcotic-acrid poisons, it may be affirmed that in large doses they act chiefly on the nervous system, in smaller doses on the alimentary canal.

Form.—Under this head will have to be considered— *a.* State of Aggregation; *b.* Chemical Combination; *c.* Mixture.

a. State of aggregation. — Solution increases the activity of poisons, both by promoting absorption and by applying them to a larger surface. Soluble poisons, therefore, are the most active, soluble salts more active than their less soluble bases, and volatile poisons act with great energy on the lungs and skin.

b. Chemical combination.—Such poisons as the mineral acids and the alkalies lose their active properties when neutralised; and as a rule, the salt resulting from the union of acid and base is more or less active in direct proportion to its solubility. Acid poisons in combining with bases, or basic poisons, combining with acids, conform to the same rule, and the resulting compounds, if soluble, retain the specific characters of their active ingredients. Thus, all the soluble salts of morphine have the same action; and the same is true of all the soluble compounds of oxalic acid. When two poisonous substances combine (as arsenious acid with copper, or prussic acid with mercury or silver), the resulting compound may give rise to the symptoms of the more active, to the mixed effects of the two, or to symptoms peculiar to itself. Lastly, some poisons insoluble in water, as arsenite of copper and carbonate of lead, or barium, may be rendered soluble and active by the acid juices of the stomach, or by the secretions of the skin.

c. Mixture.—All admixtures which render a poison more soluble make it more active; all others have a contrary effect. Thus, acids increase the activity of opium and alkaloids generally, and of the salts of copper, and water that of arsenic; but oily, mucilaginous, albuminous, and starchy liquids retard the action of poisons by protecting the coats of the stomach, by involving the poison, if in substance or powder, or even by acting as antidotes, as in the case of mercuric salts, by forming insoluble compounds. Hence the frequent escape of those who have taken large doses of arsenic or corrosive sublimate with or directly after food. Much also depends on the character of the food. Thus, arsenic in a solid dumpling would act much more slowly than in porridge, and in porridge than in liquids in common use; and strychnine in a pill more slowly than in a mixture. We avail ourselves of the protective effect of thick liquids in the treatment of cases of poisoning, and we give substances that have little power as antidotes, because they have the property of withdrawing and holding in suspension certain poisons. Powdered charcoal is the best example of this class; and magnesia and the sesquioxide of iron owe their repute as antidotes to arsenic chiefly to this property.

Part to which the poison is applied. — The effect of a poison on different parts of the body is directly as their absorbing power. Thus, poisons act most promptly when inserted into a wound; the serous surfaces hold the next place; then the stomach; then the unbroken skin. Injection into a vein insures the quickest action; but volatile poisons introduced into the lungs act nearly as promptly. The effect of the corrosive poisons and stronger irritants is proportioned to the importance of the part to which they are applied. Thus, the mineral acids prove speedily fatal when they attack the windpipe; less speedily when they act on the gullet and stomach, and they must destroy a large surface of the skin in order to kill quickly. Many animal poisons, such as those of the viper or mad dog, and also curara, introduced into the system in a minute quantity by cutaneous puncture, kill very quickly, though the same quantity, and even a much larger dose, may be swallowed with impunity.

This remarkable fact can now be physiologically explained. A certain quantity of the poison must be present in the circulation, and in the part of the body specifically affected by the poison, before it can manifest its effects; and if the excretion is as active as the absorption, no effect is produced. The poison curara is got rid of by the excretory organs as quickly as it is absorbed from the stomach. But if the excretion of urine is prevented by ligature of the renal artery, the introduction of the poison into the stomach develops its symptoms just as certainly as if it were conveyed into the circulation by a wound.

If excretion be not so rapid as absorption, the administration of small doses of the poison, which individually do not produce deleterious results, may terminate in a cumulative action with a fatal effect.

Condition of the body itself.—Under this head will have to be considered: a. Habit; b. Idiosyncrasy; c. Disease; d. Sleep.

a. Habit.—No broad general rule can be laid down as to the influence of habit. Such vegetable poisons as opium, alcohol, and tobacco, lose their effect by repetition, and may at length be taken in doses which would poison one unaccustomed to their use; but even these poisons produce permanently injurious effects; alcohol causing disease of the lungs, liver, kidneys, brain, and peripheral nerves; tobacco quickening the pulse; and opium injuring the digestion, emaciating the body, and enfeebling the mind. The less deadly mineral poisons—such as the sulphates of zinc, iron, and copper—may, however, be taken by healthy persons in continually increasing doses; even arsenic is so taken by the Styrian peasants; but arsenic, mercury, and phosphorus, when used in the arts, and gradually introduced into the system, appear, like the carbonate of lead, to be more dangerous the longer they are used. Nor do men and women who work with arsenite of copper grow more tolerant of the poison. The same effects are reproduced at each resumption of their employment.

b. Idiosyncrasy.—Under this term are included certain peculiarities of constitution, of which some may be explained by the relation between the two processes of absorption and excretion; while others cannot be satisfactorily accounted for. Idiosyncrasy may show itself in two ways—1. By difference of susceptibility without difference of action. Thus, a few grains of mercury may salivate one man, but as many drachms or ounces will not affect another. 2. By exceptional action; as when Epsom salts act like opium and opium has a purgative effect, and a simple article of diet, certain kinds of meat even mutton itself, fish, fruit, and vegetables, prove poisons to a few individuals, even when eaten in a fresh state.

c. Disease.—This, as a rule, renders the body less susceptible. Thus, patients reduced to extreme weakness by fever, are scarcely affected by stimulants which would overpower the strong. In continued and yellow fever there is great tolerance of mercury, but in paralytic affections and anæmic states an opposite condition; in anæmia large doses of steel are readily borne; and in severe dysentery, cholera, and hæmorrhage, large quantities of opium; in severe affections of the nervous system, all remedies, but especially narcotics, may be given in greatly increased doses. Delirium tremens may be safely and sucessfully treated by half-ounce doses of tincture of digitalis, and one form of mania by repeated doses of two scruples of opium. Poisons which give rise to symptoms similar to those actually existing form an exception to the rule. Thus, the irritants would increase gastritis, diarrhœa, or dysentery; and the narcotics exasperate a determination of blood to the brain, or an attack of uræmia.

d. Sleep.—In this state all the functions are languid, and the body less alive to the action of medicines and poisons. This is true of sleep artificially induced; hence, narcotics given with or before other poisons, weaken or counteract their effects. Opium, for example, when given with arsenic, not only masks the symptoms proper to that poison, but appears to retard its operation.

Classification of poisons. — Two principles of classification commend themselves as logical and useful; the one arranges poisons according to their source, the other to their action.

When the first is adopted, poisons are arranged as inorganic and organic; or as mineral, vegetable, and animal; when the second, they are grouped also in three classes—irritants, narcotics, and narcotico-irritants. To the first classification it may be objected that though most poisons from the mineral and animal kingdoms are irritants, those from the vegetable kingdom comprise, in addition to irritants, several poisons which, under any arrangement, must be distributed into many groups. On the other hand, a classification based on mode of action has the inconvenience of separating poisons which, being derived from the same kingdom of Nature, present analogies of chemical composition that render their juxtaposition extremely convenient.

By no possible classification, then, can we reconcile the conflicting requirements of physiology and natural history, or attain the highest scientific accuracy. But those who see in classification rather an instrument of convenience than an expression of abstract truth, will acquiesce in any grouping which brings into contact those objects that are best studied when they proceed or follow each other, and concerning which, when so placed, certain general principles can be laid down.

Foderé's division into irritants, narcotics, narcotico-acrids, and septics, rests on a physiological basis, as does also that which excludes the last and retains the other three. But the best toxicologists have grown dissatisfied with the third group of narcotico-acrids, and have tried to construct a classification on the same basis. The most ambitious but least successful attempt is that of Tardieu; that of Casper is scarcely an improvement; that of Dr. Taylor is less open to objection.* After examining these schemes, and the juxtapositions to which they give rise, we prefer a compromise between the claims of physiology and natural history. We first divide poisons into inorganic and organic, and then distribute them into sub-classes; the inorganic into corrosives and irritants, the organic into irritants, and such as affect the brain, spinal cord, heart, and lungs respectively; the intestinal irritation which marks the action of so many organic poisons, and justifies the use of the term narcotico-acrid, will be considered

---

* 1. Irritants et corrosifs. 2. Hyposthénisant. 3. Stupéfiants. 4. Narcotiques. 5. Nevrosthéniques. (Tardieu.) 1. Irritant poisons. 2. Poisons which produce hyperæmia. 3. Nerve paralysing poisons. 4. Poisons which produce marasmus. 5. Septic poisons. (Casper.) 1. Irritants. 2. Neurotics, distinguished as cerebral, spinal, and cerebro-spinal. (Taylor.)

as subordinate to their effect on the nervous centres, heart, and lungs. The classification, as far as it is necessary to explain it here, will therefore be as follows :—

I. **Inorganic:**
   a. Corrosive.
   b. Irritant.

II. **Organic:**
   a. Irritant.
   b. Affecting the brain, spinal cord, heart, or lungs.

CHAPTER II.

EVIDENCE OF POISONING.

AMONG the circumstances which would lead us to infer that some poison had been taken, are the **symptoms**; the **post-mortem appearances, experiments on animals, chemical analysis**, and the **conduct of suspected persons.**

Symptoms. — In most cases of poisoning the symptoms appear suddenly, in a person in good health, soon after taking food, drink, or medicine; and in most fatal cases, death happens in a few minutes, hours, or days.

The sudden appearance of the symptoms afford a presumption in favour of poisoning, for in full doses poisons act promptly. On the other hand, when given in small and repeated doses the symptoms may develop themselves gradually. But many diseases of the vital organs—brain, heart, and lungs—perforation of the stomach or intestines, and severe epidemic maladies, such as plague, cholera, yellow fever, continued fever, the febrile exanthemata, small-pox, scarlatina, and measles, and even some cases of diabetes, set in suddenly with severe and well-marked symptoms.

The occurrence of the symptoms in a person in good health also affords a presumption of poisoning; but as many acute diseases suddenly attack healthy persons, and many sudden deaths occur in others seemingly in rude health, too much stress must not be laid on this sign. It should also be borne in mind that poisons are sometimes given to the sick, and that after the health has been slowly undermined by repeated doses of some less active substance, such as tartar-emetic, death has been suddenly brought about by such deadly poisons as morphine, strychnine, or veratrine. Witness the French case of Castaign, and the English cases of Palmer, Dove, and Pritchard.

The appearance of the symptoms soon after taking food,

drink, or medicine, affords a stronger presumption : for large doses of the more active poisons act very quickly. But it must be recollected that vomiting and other symptoms of indisposition may set in after a wholesome meal ; that a full meal is a common precursor of apoplexy ; that rupture of the coats of the stomach, softened by previous disease, such as ulcer, naturally takes place while the organ is distended with food ; that English cholera may be caused by unripe fruits, putrid meat, or other unwholesome ingesta, and that a large draught of cold water, swallowed while the body is heated, may cause instant death.

The presumption afforded by the symptoms occurring soon after a meal is greatly strengthened when other persons partaking of the same meal are similarly affected ; but too much importance should not be attached to the absence of such effects in others, for the person in whom the symptoms have shown themselves may have partaken of some dish, or part of a dish, or of some wine or drink, which the others had not tasted.

The attack of several persons by similar severe symptoms, soon after a meal of which all have partaken, affords the strongest possible presumption of poisoning, either by the food itself, or by some accidental or intentional admixture.* If the symptoms are those of simple irritant poisoning, we cannot determine by the symptoms alone which of these alternatives is the true one ; but they may be so characteristic as not only to prove the administration of a poison, but to indicate the very poison itself.

The simultaneous fatal attack of several persons in the same place, or on the same mission, in the absence of proof that they had partaken of the same food, would also furnish a strong presumption of poisoning. Thus, the death in one night of four of the eight peers selected to represent the Scottish nation at the nuptials of Queen Mary with the Dauphin of France in 1558 (Lord Fleming at Paris, Bishop Reid, the Earl of Rothes, and the Earl of Cassillis

---

* When the jail-fever prevailed in England, it was not unusual to attribute to the food of which a group of persons had partaken the fatal consequences really due to the poison of the prison. In a curious case, which occurred at Redhill more than a century ago, certain Justices of the Peace all partook of the same meal, and were soon taken dangerously ill. This was at first attributed to the meal ; but the true cause (the wretched condition of a batch of paupers brought from the workhouse) was inferred from the fact that the only member of the group who had escaped, was one who had not been brought face to face with these paupers. The symptoms, as they developed themselves, confirmed the inference drawn from this exceptional occurrence.

at Dieppe), certainly justified the suspicion of poisoning, for which the refusal of the Scottish deputies to grant the crown matrimonial to the bridegroom had furnished a motive by giving great offence to the French Court.[*]

A suspicion of poisoning is often successfully rebutted by the fact that no food, drink, or medicine had been taken for hours before the commencement of an illness attributed to a quickly acting poison. The inference would be somewhat weakened if sleep had occurred in the interval.

The rapid course of the symptoms towards a fatal termination affords but a weak presumption of poisoning; for many cases of poisoning end fatally after a considerable interval, and many acute diseases run a very quick course.

All the characters now mentioned are therefore to be received with caution, and carefully weighed. The joint occurrence of two or more of them would afford a strong presumption; and the coincidence of all, though not decisive, would justify a very strong suspicion. Thus, if a person in perfect health, soon after taking food, were attacked with severe and continued vomiting and purging, and died within twenty-four hours, a strong suspicion would naturally arise that the food had contained some poisonous substance; and the suspicion would be greatly strengthened if other persons who had partaken of the same food were similarly affected. The food itself might have had poisonous properties, containing the poisonous alkaloids of putrefaction (ptomaines), or the poison might have been added to it; but the probability of poisoning in one of these two ways is very strong; and the inference would be almost irresistible if it could be shown that the person affected had never suffered in the same way before, and that neither English nor Asiatic cholera prevailed at the time.

Post-mortem appearances. — There are certain poisons and classes of poisons which leave in the dead body unmistakable signs of their action. Mineral acids stain and corrode the parts with which they come in contact, and oxalic acid in strong solution destroys and blackens the lining membrane of the gullet and stomach. Other poisons yield highly characteristic deposits. Corrosive sublimate, decomposed by the secretions and membrane of the stomach, or by its albuminous contents, leaves a slate-coloured deposit of finely divided mercury; and arsenious acid in

[*] Sharp's "Peerage"—Marquis of Ailsa.

substance a white patch clinging to the inflamed membrane, which may be changed into the yellow sulphide by sulphuretted hydrogen, the product of putrefaction. Orpiment and Scheele's green, cantharides, and nux vomica, and the spores of poisonous mushrooms also leave a coating of characteristic colour; phosphorus betrays itself by shining in the dark; and vegetable poisons are sometimes identified by seeds or fragments of leaves left in the alimentary canal.

Other poisons, again, whether inorganic or organic, both those which have a simple irritant action and those formerly classed as narcotico-acrids, excite a more intense and irregularly distributed inflammation in the stomach and intestines than that due to disease. A less degree of redness being common in those who die a natural death, would not justify a suspicion of poisoning; and the same remark applies to those appearances of congestion in the brain which are common to the action of the narcotics and narcotico-acrids, and to many cerebral diseases and disorders.

Great importance naturally attaches to the negative evidence from post-mortem appearances; such as the absence of corrosion in alleged cases of poisoning by corrosives, and of inflammation after the alleged administration of an irritant or narcotico-irritant poison. The absence of congestion of the brain in a case of imputed narcotic poisoning would afford a lower presumption.

The absence of characteristic post-mortem appearances might also become important in the very improbable event of poison being introduced into the body after death, with a view to inculpate an innocent person.

Formerly undue importance was attached to the unusual blackness or lividity of the skin, and to the early occurrence of putrefaction as evidence of poisoning. But there is no reason to believe that these appearances are more common after death by poison than after other forms of sudden or speedy death; and it is now well known that some of the mineral poisons—for instance, arsenious acid, corrosive sublimate, and chloride of zinc—preserve the parts with which they come in contact.

Post-mortem appearances similar to those produced by poison, even though confirmed by the discovery of the poison itself, would not prove that death had been caused by poison; for it might be due to some cause anticipating its fatal action. On the other hand, a dead body may bear marks of severe external injury, or extensive disease of the internal organs, and yet the real cause of death be poison.

Post-mortem appearances, then, though they furnish conclusive independent evidence in the case of several poisons, afford only a presumption in a larger number; but even when inconclusive in themselves, they may strengthen, by their presence, the presumption drawn from symptoms, or from moral evidence; or by their absence invalidate a charge prompted by malice.

Experiments on animals.—These are very valuable both as affording evidence of poisoning and as illustrating the mode of operation of poisons. Experiments, confirmed by happy accidents (as when domestic animals and poultry have partaken of the same food as the poisoned person, or have eaten the matters rejected from his stomach), have shown that the dog and cat, as well as poultry, are killed by the poisons which prove fatal to man, and that they die with symptoms similar to those by which he suffers; and when, as in poisoning by prussic acid and strychnine, the effects of the poison are quickly developed with symptoms of a very marked character, the evidence from this source must be admitted to be conclusive. But even in the absence of any previous experience of the effect of poison on a healthy living creature, its death soon after the administration of a poison which is believed to have proved fatal to a man, affords the strongest evidence in favour of his having been poisoned, even without taking into account the character of the symptoms. On the other hand, should the animal neither suffer nor die, the presumption in favour of the harmlessness of the substance under trial is very strong. When the substance supposed to contain poison is so abundant that it can be given to different animals, or when the matters rejected from the stomach happen to be eaten by them, the death of all the animals affords undoubted proof of poisoning.

In rare cases of poisoning of animals by arsenic or strychnine, good evidence has been afforded by the fatal effect on other animals of eating their flesh.

The value of the evidence from experiments on animals is affected by certain considerations arising out of the discrepant effects of the same poison on different living creatures. It has been ascertained beyond all doubt that there is at least one insect that can feed and flourish on strychnine; and nearly half a century ago, M. Runge, of Berlin, fed a rabbit exclusively for no less than eight days on the leaves of belladonna, hyoscyamus, and stramonium, and though he found that the poisonous principles had been taken up into the animal's body, the animal at the end of the time was as healthy as at the beginning; there was not even any dilatation of the pupil. Dr. W. Ogle, in a letter addressed to the *Times* in August 1865, applies this fact to the case of Mr. Sprague, tried for attempting to poison the Chalker family, and acquitted; and deems it probable that the belladonna found its way into the poisoned pie through the flesh of a rabbit which had fed on the plant. This explanation must be admitted to be feasible; for it has been well ascertained that poisonous plants, which prove harmless to insects, birds, and animals that use or consume them, may impart to their secretions and flesh properties highly poisonous to human beings. Thus, the honey of bees collected from the calmia, azalea, and rhododendron, and even the mead made from them, has been found poisonous. During the famous retreat of the 10,000 under Xenophon the army suffered severely by eating the honey collected from the Azalea pontica. The milk, as well as the flesh, of cattle browsing on some of the herbage in South America has proved poisonous; as has the flesh of hares that had eaten the Rhododendron chrysanthemum, that of pheasants that had fed on the buds and shoots of the Calmia latifolia, and that of partridges that had partaken of certain berries during the Canadian winter, and had been imported into this country packed in ice; in September 1862, Mr. F. Taylor, of Romsey, reported two cases of great severity from eating the Canadian partridge, and the case of a cat sickened and paralysed by the same cause, and in the same year several persons near Toulouse were poisoned by a dish of snails fattened on the leaves and shoots of Coriaria myrtifolia.*

It may be safely conceded, therefore, that certain poisons belonging to the vegetable kingdom may be consumed with impunity by insects, birds, and mammals, and yet the honey collected by bees, the flesh of birds, and the milk and flesh of animals, if consumed by human beings, may occasion distinct, dangerous, and even fatal symptoms of poisoning.

To the evidence drawn from experiments on animals with matters rejected from the human stomach, or collected from the stomach and intestines after death, it has been objected that the

* *Med. Times and Gaz.*, Sept. 13, 1862.

animal secretions may be so vitiated as themselves to prove poisonous, and the objection has been enforced by a well-known experiment of Morgagni. The bile from the stomach of a child, who died in convulsions from tertian ague, mixed with bread and given to a cock, caused convulsions and death in a few minutes, and the same effect followed in two pigeons inoculated with it. But it is obvious that experiments with the bile of a diseased subject can have no proper application to cases in which food rejected from a healthy stomach has proved poisonous to animals.

It is scarcely necessary to state that the negative result of experiments with substances rejected from the stomach, or found there after death, is not conclusive against poisoning, for the poisonous substance may have been evaporated, decomposed, absorbed, or previously rejected.

When there is reason to believe that we are dealing with a small quantity of poison, small animals, such as rats or mice, should be chosen for experiment; or the frog, as particularly adapted for experiment with minute quantities of such poisons as strychnine. The hypodermic method of administering such active medicines as morphine and coniïne will evidently admit of extension to the identification of poisonous substances, as soon as sufficient data have been collected by well-devised experiments.*

The necessity of experiments on animals is now largely superseded by chemical analysis; but as the tests for some of the vegetable poisons are uncertain, such experiments, performed with care, are valuable, and have been admitted as evidence; † as a rule, they are more delicate than chemical investigation.

When experiments on animals are resorted to in order to illustrate the mode of operation of poisons, or to determine some important question, such as the shortest time within which a dose of prussic acid may prove fatal, or the possible absence of marks of inflammation in the stomach after poisoning by some irritant, such as corrosive sublimate, choice should be made of the dog, as the animal of which we have the largest experience.

Chemical analysis.—This form of evidence, though not

* Dr. John Harley's Gulstonian Lectures, given at the College of Physicians (1868).

† By the Cruelty to Animals Act, 1876, any Judge of the Superior Courts is empowered to grant a licence for such experiments if he should think them desirable in a criminal case.

absolutely necessary when the symptoms, post-mortem appearances, and circumstantial evidence confirm each other, or even when two of the three coincide, is always of the first importance. The poison may be discovered in the living person by tests applied to the urine, to the blood abstracted by bleeding, cupping, or leeches, or to the serum of a blistered surface; or it may be detected in the dead body in the blood, flesh, viscera, and secretions. In either case the discovery of a poison affords conclusive evidence of its administration.

When we are dealing with substances rejected from the stomach or voided by the bowels, with the contents of the stomach and bowels after death, or with food or medicine of which the sufferer has partaken, the evidence is obviously less conclusive, for objections may be raised on each of the three suppositions, that poison is detected, that it is not detected, or that it is found in very small quantity.

When a poison is found in the matters discharged during life, or left in the alimentary canal after death, or in food or medicine, it may be objected that it might have been accidentally mixed with it, or fraudulently, in order to inculpate an innocent party; in which case the evidence must be supported by proof that this could not have happened. In this connection, too, the subject of the alkaloids produced by putrefaction must be taken into account.

But when a poison is not found in any of the substances submitted to analysis, it does not follow that none has been taken; for, in the case of a meal actually containing poison, and followed by symptoms of poisoning, the articles submitted to analysis may not contain the poison, though some other portion of the meal may. The poison may even be so unequally distributed through a single dish that the part examined may not contain it, though other parts of it do. The poison may be in the gravy, and not in the meat; or it may have been sprinkled only on the outside of the joint. Again, we may fail to detect poison in the contents of the stomach and intestines, because it had been rejected or evacuated, absorbed, decomposed, or evaporated; or because it belongs to that large class of vegetable poisons which we have not yet found the means of discovering with certainty. Poisons are most likely to be rejected or evacuated when they belong to the class of irritants absorbed when they are in a fluid state or soluble, decomposed when they belong to the animal or vegetable kingdom. Poisons which are insoluble, or sparingly soluble, such as arsenic, may often be detected in the stomach, and sometimes in the intestines, after repeated vomiting and purging, being glued to the mucous coat by the tenacious products of inflammation.

When the examination of the body is delayed, and in cases of disinterment, we may fail to discover a poison which was in the body at the time of death, from its having exuded through the textures, evaporated, or been decomposed. This observation does not apply to mineral poisons; for though subject to change by the decay of the textures, they are transformed, not destroyed. Thus, arsenious acid may be converted into the yellow sulphide; and corrosive sublimate may be changed into the black sulphide of mercury, or to calomel, by contact with the mucous membrane, or it may deposit finely divided mercury. Among animal poisons, cantharides, and among vegetable poisons, strychnine, may be mentioned as undergoing little or no change from the decay of the textures.

It is scarcely necessary to add that malicious or mistaken imputations of poisoning may be shown to be unfounded by the non-discovery of poisons in the matters alleged to contain it.

When poison is found in very small quantity, the objection is sure to be advanced, that it was not enough to account for death; but to this the reply is obvious, that the quantity found must needs fall short of that actually taken; for it is always only a part of the matter vomited or otherwise expelled from the body, of the contents of the alimentary canal after death, or of the blood, tissues, or viscera of the body, which is submitted to analysis, and that the quantity found in the stomach is only the surplus of what may have been sufficient to cause death by absorption. The discovery, therefore, of a quantity of poison insufficient to destroy life is scarcely even a presumption that the substance was not administered in a poisonous dose, though it is consistent with the supposition that it had been given as a medicine.

But the value of chemical analysis as evidence of poisoning is not limited to the discovery of a poison by a single analysis; for by comparing one analysis with another, important light may be thrown on the mode of administration, and the innocence or guilt of a suspected or accused party. A bowl of porridge, eaten at breakfast by a female believed to have died poisoned, was found to contain arsenic. The chemical analysis showed that the poison was not mixed with the store of meal, but only with the part used in making the porridge; and as other circumstances justified the inference that the poison had been mixed with the meal in the morning before any stranger entered the house, the husband (the only other inmate) was convicted of the murder. In the case of an opposite kind, arsenic was found mixed with a large mass of flour, as well as with the part used in making bread. It was accordingly inferred that the flour had been ground from wheat intended for seed mixed with arsenic to destroy insects, and sent in mistake to the mill.*

In several cases of poisoning by corrosive acids the clothes of the suspected murderer have been stained in the same way as the clothes and body of his victim.

The cases just referred to are examples of qualitative analysis. The value which may sometimes attach to quantitative analysis is shown by the two cases which follow.

Mr. Hodgson, a surgeon, was tried at Durham in 1824 for attempting to poison his wife. He had substituted corrosive sublimate for calomel in opium pills, prescribed by her physician, but this he said, was a mistake committed while he was intoxicated. It was also proved to have been contained in a laudanum draught ordered by her physician; but this, too, as he alleged, was an injection of corrosive sublimate previously prepared for a sailor, but which he had taken for a water-bottle. But on submitting the draught and the injection to chemical analysis, the former was found to contain fourteen grains, while the latter contained only five grains to the ounce.†

Samuel Whalley was indicted at York Spring Assizes in 1821 for administering arsenic to Martha King, pregnant by him; but of the tarts in which the arsenic was alleged to have been administered, the portions eaten could not have contained more than ten grains, while the matters alleged to have been vomited contained, even after repeated vomiting, fifteen grains.

Conduct of suspected persons.—Great importance is very properly attached, in trials for poisoning, to the conduct of the prisoner before, during, and after the illness of the deceased. He

---

* Cases quoted from Alison and Barruel by Christison, "On Poisons," p. 75.

† For a full report of this interesting case, see the *Edin. Med. and Surg. Journal,* vol. xxii. p. 438.

is often proved, without adequate motive, to have made a study of poisons and their properties, and to have purchased them under false pretences; to have compounded medicine or prepared food for the deceased; to have sought opportunities of administering them; to have made himself the sole attendant on the deceased; to have kept near relatives and other inconvenient witnesses at a distance; to have placed obstacles in the way of obtaining proper medical assistance; to have made hurried arrangements for the funeral; to have opposed the examination of the body; to have hastily disposed of matters which might have been examined; to have tampered with the matters reserved for analysis. Such acts as these, some of which are likely to fall under the notice of a medical attendant, will have to be carefully weighed by the jury, together with such other items of general or circumstantial evidence as point to the existence of an obvious motive or inducement to the crime, or indicate the previous state of mind of the deceased as affording a probability, or the reverse, of suicide.

Symptoms and post-mortem appearances proper to the different classes of poisons.—There are two classes of poisons which present both symptoms and post-mortem appearances of a well-defined character—the corrosives and the irritants, and a third class, divided into important sub-classes, according as they affect the brain, the spinal cord, the heart, or the lungs, in which the symptoms are well-marked, but the post-mortem appearances less constant, the alimentary canal being subject to like uncertainty of action and post-mortem appearance. This third class formerly comprised the two distinct divisions of narcotics and narcotico-acrids.

a. **Corrosives.**—This class of poisons is characterised, as the name implies, by their destructive action on the parts with which they come in contact. If they were to act on a large extent of the cutaneous surface, they would destroy life as burns and scalds of like extent and severity. When swallowed, they prove fatal by the same destructive action on the lining membrane of the alimentary canal or of the windpipe, the immediate causes of death being shock, exhaustion, perforation of the stomach or intestines, starvation from stricture of the gullet, or extensive destruction of the secreting membrane of the stomach, and in rare cases, occurring chiefly in young children, suffocation from injury to the glottis and windpipe. These effects are produced, among inorganic poisons, by the mineral acids and the caustic alkalies and their carbonates; among the organic poisons by strong solutions of oxalic acid and of tartaric and citric acids. In the group of inorganic poisons there are also several corrosive soluble salts (chlorides) of the metals mercury, antimony, zinc, and tin, which combine with their direct corrosive action remote specific effects in addition to the remote reflex effect of the corrosion itself.

The *symptoms* due to these poisons are well marked. They have a strong acid, alkaline, or metallic taste, and cause a burning pain, which occurs almost simultaneously in the mouth, throat, gullet, and stomach, whence it extends rapidly to the entire abdomen. This is soon followed by vomiting, and after no long interval by purging. The matters discharged contain blood, either unchanged or decomposed by the poison. The epiglottis and upper part of the windpipe are often so corroded as to occasion suffocation and speedy death.

The *post-mortem appearances* are those of corrosion, mixed with corrugation from strong contraction of the muscular fibres, and followed by inflammation and its consequences. The corrosions may be confined to small spots, or may extend over a large surface; may be limited to a removal of portions, more or less considerable, of the lining membrane of the gullet and stomach, or may destroy all their coats, so as to occasion perforations large or small, and the discharge of considerable portions of the organs themselves (as well as of casts of them resulting from the action of the acids on their secretions) by vomiting or by stool. Beyond the corroded parts the textures are acutely inflamed, sometimes gangrenous, often black from blood extravasated into the cellular tissue beneath, or injection of the vessels with dark blood. Sometimes the tissues are found softened, sometimes hardened and shrivelled. These poisons often produce in the gullet a peculiar wrinkled and worm-eaten appearance, due to the contraction of the longitudinal and transverse fibres, and the removal of patches of epithelium. (See Figs. 62, 63, and 64, p. 481.)

As these effects of the corrosive poisons may possibly be mistaken for post-mortem appearances due to other causes, it may be well to point out more particularly the characters by which the one may be distinguished from the other.

Softening of the mucous membrane due to the corrosives is attended by changes of colour, arising, in the case of the mineral acids, from their direct action on the tissues, in the case of corrosive sublimate, from the deposit of the finely divided metal or its sulphide. In the case of some other corrosive poisons we are not assisted by these changes, but must be guided by the state of the gullet and the action on the skin and clothes. The hardened and crimped state of the parts with which the corrosive comes in contact is eminently characteristic; it is never present in disease. The black injection of the vessels is not conclusive, for it may be produced by the action of any acid liquid or the acid secretion of the stomach itself. Gangrene is a rare result of disease, and the black infiltration into the submucous tissue for which it is sometimes mistaken is equally uncommon. Ulceration and consequent perforation, the result of the action of the corrosives, is to be distinguished, in the case of most of them, by characteristic colours; and this is true both of small ulcers and of extensive destruction of the tissues. The characters of ulcers from disease will be presently described when speaking of irritant poisons. The extensive destruction of the coats that sometimes arises from the action of the gastric juice after death belongs to this place.

The destructive action of the gastric juice after death was formerly a subject of controversy; but the fact of its sometimes taking place has been placed beyond a doubt by observations in man and experiments on animals. The usual seat of the opening is the posterior part of the stomach, but it varies with the position of the body. The aperture may be as small as a shilling or as large as the palm of the hand; and it has even been found to occupy one-half of the stomach. It may assume any shape; its edges are fringed, softened, and smeared with a dark pulpy mass; and the vessels of the stomach are often found injected with dark blood—a common action, as already stated, of acid fluids. The neighbouring viscera sometimes undergo a similar change. Occasionally there is more than one aperture. As there is no inflammation around the opening, it is not possible to confound this post-mortem change with the effect of an irritant poison, which would be attended by marks of acute inflammation, and by characteristic stains and deposits. When the gastric juice acts only on the mucous membrane of the stomach, it gives it a soft gelatinous appearance of a black or dark-brown colour.

Perforation of the intestines is very rare in cases of corrosive poisoning, and perforation of the gullet still less common. Both may occur from diseases not difficult to recognise after death.

b. **Irritant poisons.**—Substances that inflame the parts to which they are applied are said to act as irritants to those parts; and those which produce the same effect on the alimentary canal are also termed irritants: and, with the exceptions indicated when defining the term poison, of hot and cold water, and such articles as pins, needles, and powdered glass, may claim admission into the list of irritant poisons, if they prove in any instance fatal to life, or produce symptoms of great severity.

The class of irritants comprises mineral, animal, and vegetable substances; it contains a greater number of individual poisons than all the remaining classes put together; and it also contributes largely to the list of cases of poisoning. It accounts for nearly one-fourth of the annual deaths from ascertained poisons, of which the great majority are metallic irritants.

Of this large class, two groups admit of distinction and separation; one, the members of which destroy life by irritating the parts to which they are applied; the other, by adding to local irritation peculiar or specific remote effects. To the first group belong the principal vegetable irritants, some of the alkaline salts used in medicine, the less active metallic poisons, some products of destructive distillation, and the irritant gases. The second group comprises the metallic irritants—arsenic, mercury, antimony, lead, and copper; the metalloidal elements, phosphorus and iodine; and one product of the animal kingdom, cantharides.

The *symptoms* caused by irritant poisons, as a class, are burning pain and constriction in the throat and gullet; sharp pain, increased by pressure, in the pit of the stomach, intense thirst, nausea and vomiting, followed by pain, tension, and tenderness of the entire abdomen, and purging attended with tenesmus, and frequently with dysuria. The constitutional symptoms vary with the intensity of the irritation and the interval which has elapsed since the administration of the poison, being at one time those of collapse, at another of inflammatory fever. The mode of death also varies. One patient will not rally from the first shock to the nervous system; a second dies in strong convulsions; a third worn out by protracted suffering; a fourth starved through the permanent injury inflicted on the gullet and stomach.

These symptoms vary in severity, and in the time and order of their occurrence, with the quantity of the poison, its solubility, and the full or empty state of the stomach. When the poison is sparingly soluble, as is the case with arsenious acid, the pain and sense of constriction in the throat and gullet are not felt immediately on swallowing it, but after an interval more or less considerable, and occasionally they are absent, or they follow the other symptoms instead of preceding them, in consequence of the repeated contact of the dissolved or suspended poison with the upper portions of the tube, in the act of vomiting. The stronger and more soluble irritant poisons cause the discharges to be mixed with blood, which happens rarely, and to a less extent, in the case of the simple irritants, and they sometimes inflame the upper part of the windpipe, giving rise to hoarseness, wheezing respiration, and harassing cough, occasionally ending in suffocation.

The *post-mortem appearances* caused by the irritants are those of inflammation and its consequences.

The simple irritants give rise to inflammation more or less severe, followed by its usual consequences. In some cases there is merely increased vascularity, in others deep redness; and the surface may be coated with a tenacious secretion, and the cavity filled with a glairy mucus. The coats may be found thickened through the intensity of the inflammation, black from bloody extravasation into the submucous tissue, ulcerated, gangrenous, and sloughing, softened, but occasionally hard and shrivelled. Vessels filled with dark blood are sometimes found ramifying minutely over the surface, which in other instances is studded with black points. These appearances are not confined to the stomach, but are found in the fauces and gullet, and in the duodenum. The rest of the small intestines is often the seat of acute inflammation, with ulceration and softening of the mucous membrane; ulcers are also found in the large intestines and excoriation of the anus. In some cases the lining membrane of the larynx and air passages is inflamed.

Several of these symptoms and post-mortem appearances are not peculiar to poisoning; they may be present in English and Asiatic cholera, in acute inflammation of the stomach or bowels, in rupture of these parts, or of other viscera of the abdomen. They may also be produced by drinking hot or cold water; and authors have been at some pains to show that simple distension of the stomach, vomiting and purging of blood, colic, strangulated hernia, obstruction of the bowels, diarrhœa, and dysentery, have some symptoms in common with ordinary cases of irritant poisoning, and may still more nearly resemble certain exceptional cases. Though some of the objections founded on this possible resemblance of disease to poisoning are of little force, it may be well to point out some leading features in which the diseases in question differ from the usual effects of irritant poisons.

In English cholera the evacuations very rarely contain blood, and there is no pain and constriction in the throat, though there may be some soreness as the result of constant efforts to vomit. The disease prevails chiefly in summer and autumn, and is rarely fatal, except in children. In Asiatic cholera, too, discharge of blood is a very rare occurrence, though the evacuations sometimes have a port wine tint; and the pain and constriction of the throat are wanting. In both diseases the purging follows the vomiting much more rapidly than in cases of poisoning. There is one group of cases of poisoning by arsenic in which the symptoms so nearly resemble those of two forms of cholera that medical men have fallen into error without seriously affecting their reputation. Acute inflammation of the stomach, except as the result of drinking hot or cold water, or as the effect of some irritant substance not esteemed poisonous, is very rare, and is not attended by pain and constriction of the throat, or by diarrhœa. Acute inflammation of the bowels affects their peritoneal covering, and is attended with constipation. Distension of the stomach, though an occasional cause of severe suffering and of sudden death, does not admit of being mistaken for the effect of a class of poisons of which vomiting is a leading symptom. Indeed, a full stomach is in itself the strongest possible presumption against irritant poisoning. Rupture of the stomach, occurring, as it often does, during or directly after a meal, and through an effort to vomit, followed by sudden and violent pain, by collapse, and by death instantly, or in from four or five to less than twenty-four hours, might naturally raise a suspicion of poisoning, which nothing short of a post-mortem examination could set at rest. The same observation applies to rupture of the inner coat alone (a very rare occurrence) and to rupture of the intestines or other viscera of the abdomen, all of which accidents may be followed by vomiting with excruciating pain, and extreme tenderness of the abdomen, cold skin, feeble pulse, and symptoms of collapse with death within twenty-four hours. The effect of drinking hot water differs from that of the simple corrosives chiefly in the absence of characteristic stains, and the negative result of an analysis. The drinking of cold liquids sometimes causes vomiting and purging, and other symptoms allied to those of irritant poisoning ; and in the absence of a complete history of the case we may have to resort to the negative evidence afforded by the result of an analysis.

Of vomiting and purging of blood it will be sufficient to remark that they are not accompanied by urgent symptoms suggestive of the action of poison ; of diarrhœa and dysentery that, in the great majority of cases of poisoning, discharges from the bowels are associated with vomiting, and of colic, strangulated hernia, and obstruction of the bowels that they are attended by constipation, and that the vomited matters are often feculent.

The post-mortem appearances in irritant poisoning are not always characteristic, and it is true of the more common appearances, as of some of the more usual symptoms, that they may be occasioned by disease. Those usually specified are (1) **Redness;** (2) **Gangrene and lividity;** (3) **Softening;** (4) **Ulceration;** and (5) **Perforation of the mucous membrane.**

(1) **Redness of the mucous membrane.**—This may be produced by colouring matter ; but when it is due to blood contained in the vessels, it may be traced to subsidence after death, to repletion of the small vessels by the contraction of the arteries, to transudation through the peritoneal covering of the liver or spleen, to congestion in cases of sudden death, especially if caused by asphyxia, when it often occurs in large bright patches, or lastly, it may result from the flow of blood to the stomach which accompanies digestion. Sometimes, too, a remarkable redness of the stomach is found after death, without any symptoms having occurred during life to account for it. Hence, mere redness of the mucous coat of the stomach is not to be regarded as a proof of inflammation ; but when it is combined with softening, putrefaction not having set in ; when the membrane itself is covered with a thick and tenacious mucus, when it it opaque, so that when dissected off it hides the finger over which it is stretched, the redness may certainly be attributed to inflammation. The same remarks apply to the intestines.

(2) **Gangrene and lividity.**—Gangrene of the mucous membrane is a well-known consequence of obstructed circulation in cases of hernia, and of internal constriction, and authors of reputation

have described it as a consequence of acute inflammation; but it is probable that infiltrated blood blackened by acid secretions has been often confounded with it.

Lividity.—A minute injection of the vessels with black blood (Figs. 64, 65, pp. 481, 482), may result from the action of an acid introduced from without, or generated within the body; and it can be produced after death by pouring any of the mineral acids into the intestines. Lividity or blackness, then, when not caused by gangrene, is not due to disease, but is the effect of some acid, swallowed or secreted. The blackness sometimes met with in the intestines in acute dysentery and enteritis, if not gangrenous, is probably due to the same cause. The deposit of black pigment known as melanosis, is distinguished by being arranged in regular, well-defined spots, without thickening of the membrane or signs of surrounding inflammation.

(3) Softening.—The mucous membrane may be softened or hardened by the action of poisons, or as the result of inflammation caused by them; or it results from disease, and it is a very common effect of the action of the gastric juice after death. Softening due to the action of the non-corrosive irritants is attended by marks of acute inflammation, but as a rule morbid softening is not preceded by any characteristic symptoms.

(4) Ulceration.—Ulcers of the stomach may be caused by disease or by poison. Those caused by disease are the cancerous ulcer, the chronic ulcer, and the tubercular. It is difficult to mistake the ulcer of cancer for that caused by poisoning; the presence of a tumour and the microscopical characters at once deciding the point. The chronic ulcer varies in size from a fourpenny piece to half-a-crown. It is round or oval, and when recent it appears as if punched out of the mucous membrane of the stomach, with little, if any, surrounding congestion; it may penetrate all the coats of the stomach, the size of the ulceration diminishing in each coat, so that the ulcer is conical, with the apex outwards. When old, the edges are thickened, sometimes greatly and externally; there are adhesions of the peritoneum to surrounding parts. More than one-third of the ulcers occupy the posterior surface of the stomach, more than three-fourths either that part, the lesser curvature, or the neighbourhood of the pylorus. The ulcers caused by poisoning are the result of a more intense inflammation; and they are often found discoloured, as in the case of poisoning by nitric acid,

and iodine; or covered with a white powder, as in poisoning by arsenic; or coated with the decomposed poison, such as the black powder (minutely divided mercury) formed by the decomposition of corrosive sublimate, or the yellow sulphide of arsenic formed during the process of putrefaction after death.

(5) **Perforation of the stomach.**—This may arise from—1. Corrosion; 2. Inflammation, followed by ulceration; 3. Chronic gastric ulcer; and 4. The action of the gastric juice after death.

1. Perforation from corrosion.—It is impossible, as already stated, to confound a perforation due to the action of a corrosive poison with any perforation arising from natural causes acting either during life or after death, The state of the mouth, throat, and gullet, and often of the skin and clothes of the deceased, renders the distinction easy; and in many cases the contents of the stomach or bowels escape into the cavity of the abdomen, and leave traces of their action on other viscera.

2. Perforation from ulceration, the result of irritant poisoning, is very rare.

3. Perforation from chronic ulcer of the stomach is not a rare affection. It is not an infrequent occurrence in young females from fifteen to twenty-five years of age, and often after slight symptoms of indisposition. The rupture generally takes place soon after a meal, more rarely as a consequence of sudden exertion, and it is instantly followed by sharp pain of the abdomen, and symptoms of acute peritoneal inflammation. There is little vomiting, and no purging; the patient dies in a state of collapse in from eighteen to thirty-six hours; but in some cases, when the stomach is nearly empty, the fatal event is postponed, the inflammation being of limited extent or subacute in character. The opening in the peritoneum is generally small, and the ulcer has the peculiar characters just described.* The absence of marks of acute inflammation and of characteristic discolorations, the non-detection of poison in the stomach or in the contents of the abdomen, the sudden occurrence of pain in the belly as the first symptom, the slight vomiting, and the absence of diarrhœa distinguish this form of perforation from that due to poison.

4. The destruction and consequent perforation caused by the gastric juice after death has already been spoken of at p. 440.

---

* Consult Brinton "On the Pathology, Symptoms, and Treatment of Ulcer of the Stomach"; and Taylor's Essay in *Guy's Hospital Reports*, No. 8.

c. **Poisons neither Corrosives nor Irritants.**—The poisons which are neither corrosives nor irritants, or which, if they act in either of these ways, prove fatal by their effect on the nerve centres, and through them on the heart or lungs, were formerly comprised under the two heads of narcotics and narcotico-acrids, oxalic acid (a corrosive in strong solution) being the principal exception. These two classes are now more conveniently treated in different sections, according as their most obvious and striking symptoms, when given in full doses and acting in their usual manner, are those of the brain, spinal cord, heart, or lungs. They will be grouped, for the sake of convenience, as affecting the brain, spinal cord, heart, and lungs respectively. This arrangement is based on some notable prevailing symptom, or group of symptoms ; not on the precise *modus operandi* or proximate and real cause of death.

1. The poisons which affect the brain may be distributed into three leading sub-classes ; one group, of which opium is the type, causing sleep more or less profound ; a second, of which belladonna is the type, producing delirium, with illusions ; and a third, of which alcohol is the type, giving rise to exhilaration, followed by delirium or sleep, or both successively or alternately, according to the dose and the constitution of the individual.

The group of poisons of which opium is the most conspicuous member, owes its importance less to the number of individuals which it comprises (for they are few), than to the habitual use made of them by large classes of persons, their constant employment in the treatment of medical and surgical maladies, the many accidents to which they give rise, and the many occasions on which they are employed by the suicide and murderer. Opium and its preparations alone are taken in nearly half the cases in which the poison can be identified.

The poisons of this sub-class presents difficulties which do not occur in the case of irritants. Their symptoms more nearly resemble those of disease, and the post-mortem appearances are often indistinct, and, even when best marked, not highly characteristic. The chemical analysis also is less sure and satisfactory than in the case of irritant poisoning. The symptoms proper to this class are giddiness, headache, dimness of sight, extreme contraction of the pupil, noises in the ears, drowsiness and confusion of mind, passing into insensibility more or less complete. Delirium is rare, and paralysis, convulsions, and tetanic spasms only of occasional occurrence. There is no direct irritation of the stomach and bowels, but nausea and vomiting may occur, not at the commencement (as in the case of irritants), but when the patient begins to recover. Diarrhœa also is a rare incident. The post-mortem appearances consist in fulness of the veins and sinuses of the brain, effusion of serum beneath the membranes at the base, or into the ventricles; and, in a few cases, extravasation of blood.

There are several diseases of the nerve centres, which, in common with opium and its preparations, have coma more or less profound, and insensibility more or less complete, as prominent symptoms. Cerebral hæmorrhage and congestion, hydrocephalus, blows and injuries of the head, febrile affections in certain stages, uræmia and acetonæmia, the close of an epileptic fit, exposure to extreme cold, and many poisons in certain stages of their action, are attended by a profound sleep, from which the patient is not easily roused, or even with coma and insensibility. The diagnosis of disease and poisoning during life will therefore sometimes be difficult, especially in infants and young children; and after death the appearances of the brain may prove inconclusive. The discovery of disease of the kidney would furnish a probability of uræmia, and inflammation or chronic disease of the brain, or any considerable collection of serum upon or within it, would supply a sufficient explanation of death.

The sub-class of poisons of which belladonna is the best example is strongly characterised by delirium, spectral illusions, and a largely dilated pupil, with dryness of mouth and throat and thirst, without any characteristic post-mortem appearance. Tetanic spasms, heightened sensibility, paralysis of the motor and sensory nerves, coma, and insensibility, are among the exceptional symptoms; but great difference in degree, and strange varieties in the combination of these elements are observed in different cases of poisoning by the same substance. It must also be borne in mind that the delirium which is the leading symptom of the group is also a symptom often present in fevers and febrile disorders, and generally in diseases or injuries attended or followed by fever. Illusions also which are present in this form of poisoning are occasioned by many different and by some trivial causes.

The poisons of this class owe their active properties each to one well-defined active principle (atropine and hyoscyamine), but they are commonly taken in the form of leaves, berries, seeds, or root;

and these, or portions of them, may often be identified in the contents of the alimentary canal rejected during life or found there after death. When intestinal irritation is added to the other symptoms, it is due to such solid matters, and not to these active principles.

The third sub-class of poisons, of which alcohol is the type, is characterised rather by the succession or combination of the symptoms, than by any one dominant symptom. Excitement of circulation and of the cerebral functions, passing into muscular weakness, shown by want of power as well as by want of co-ordination of movement and by double vision, and this into profound sleep, coma, and insensibility, constitute the usual group and succession of symptoms. Excitement followed by somnolency, and excitement culminating in maniacal violence, are not uncommon.

The more chronic form of poisoning by this class is characterised by tremor, delirium, and illusions, and the other symptoms of the disease known as delirium tremens.

It should be borne in mind that the ordinary effects of alcohol may show themselves as a result of the action of extreme cold, and that they are sometimes present in the early stages of some mental disorders. The presence or absence of the odour of the poison in the breath of the patient greatly assists the diagnosis.

2. The poisons which affect the spinal cord consist chiefly of strychnine and the plants which yield it. The tetanic spasms which it occasions constitute the leading symptom and sign of their action, and these are present also in tetanus, traumatic and idiopathic, and exceptionally, as one of several symptoms, in poisoning by many of the more active narcotics of every class. The differences between poisoning and disease will be indicated elsewhere.

3. The poisons which affect the heart kill either by sudden shock or by syncope or collapse less rapidly induced. The first division comprises hydrocyanic acid and the substances that contain it, and oxalic acid and its salts. The second embraces aconite, digitalis, tobacco, lobelia inflata, veratrine, and some poisons of less importance. A knowledge of their characteristic symptoms may be important in cases of sudden and speedy death. In the case of hydrocyanic acid we are happily greatly assisted by its characteristic odour; in poisoning by oxalic acid, by its corrosive action on the gullet and stomach; and in that of aconite, by its peculiar effect on the lips, tongue, and palate.

4. The poisons which act on the lungs, and so destroy life, have for their type carbonic acid gas, which occasions the symptoms and post-mortem appearances present in death by asphyxia, however brought about. The operation of this class may have to be distinguished from asphyxia produced by other causes; and it should be well understood that in poisoning by many of the more active poisons, and notably by prussic acid in doses short of a quickly fatal one, life may be destroyed by a remote action on the lungs, producing fatal asphyxia.

CHAPTER III.

METHODS OF PROCEDURE IN CASES OF POISONING.

THE facts and discussions of the preceding chapter have prepared the way for a more direct examination of the duties that devolve on the medical man in cases of alleged poisoning.

Suspicion of poisoning may arise under very different circumstances. It may spring up in the minds of persons ignorant of the nature and action of poisons, suggested by some severe illness or sudden or speedy death, coupled with the suspicious conduct of some relative or friend; or it may occur to the medical man himself during his attendance on a patient; or, again, it may be the utterly groundless fancy of a person of unsound mind, such fancy constituting the leading feature of his malady, or one only of his many delusions. But in whatever way the medical man may be brought to entertain and consider a suspicion of poisoning, the following summary of the leading circumstances to be attended to and noted down, cannot fail to be of service.

1. **The patient.**—The state of the patient before the commencement of the symptoms, whether in good health or suffering from illness; the time at which they began, and at what interval after a meal, or after taking food, drink, or medicine; their nature, order, and time of occurrence, and the period of the commencement of any new symptom or train of symptoms: whether they followed the use of any new article of food or medicine; increased steadily in severity, or alternated with intervals of ease; and whether the exacerbations corresponded with a repetition of food or medicine, also the character of any substances which may have been rejected from the stomach or passed from the bowels. The exact time of the death should be noted, and, if the person is found dead, when he was last seen alive.

2. **Food and Medicine.**—If the symptoms of poisoning showed

themselves soon after a meal, minute inquiries should be made as to the cooking of the several dishes; the vessels used in the preparation of the food should be inspected, and their contents, if necessary, preserved; and suspicious powders or liquids found in the house should be sealed and kept. If several persons have partaken of the same meal, care should be taken to ascertain what articles were taken by those who suffered and by those who escaped, and in what quantities, and whether the same articles of food had been previously taken without bad effect by the persons attacked.

3. **The ejecta.**—The vomited matters must be carefully collected, and removed from the clothing, furniture, &c., on which they had been ejected; and portions of the dress, furniture, or flooring may, if necessary, be reserved for examination.

4. **Post-mortem examination.**—But suspicions of poisoning may first occur to the medical man during a post-mortem examination, or he may be required to make such an examination in consequence of suspicions having already arisen in the minds of relatives, or in the course of an inquiry in the coroner's court. In certain cases, too, he may be required to conduct the disinterment as well as the post-mortem examination of a body supposed to contain poison. Hence the importance to the medical man of being furnished with a summary of rules and suggestions to guide him in this important and responsible duty.

Having observed the precautions insisted on at p. 276 as common to all post-mortem examinations for legal purposes, certain others proper to cases of suspected poisoning will have to be taken. These arise out of the fact that while poisons themselves, as well as their most notable effects, are found in the alimentary canal, they, and certain of their secondary effects, are to be sought after in the organs and tissues into which they are carried by the blood. The alimentary canal and the principal viscera, or parts of them, and in some cases blood or portions of muscle, will have to be set aside for more minute examination; and they may have to be forwarded to some skilful chemist for analysis, unless the person making the post-mortem feels himself competent to the task.

Prior to the inspection, one large wide-mouthed jar, of glass or earthenware, and a few smaller ones, should be got ready, which, if not new, should be repeatedly washed out with water and drained, so as to be quite clean. They should be furnished with clean ground-glass stoppers, or with new corks, or other non-metallic means of closure. The larger jar is for the intestinal canal and its contents ; the smaller for the other viscera, or parts of them. The method of procedure, as far as it relates to the intestinal canal, must be governed by such considerations as the following :—When the poison is a corrosive its effects are to be looked for chiefly in the mouth, tongue, throat, windpipe, gullet, stomach, and upper part of the small intestines ; and, in case of perforation, in the contents of the peritoneum. But if the poison is one of those irritants which combine local action with remote specific effects, we may find marks of its direct action on the gullet, stomach, small intestines, and even on the whole intestinal canal ; while the viscera to which it is carried with the blood may also become inflamed, and especially those engaged in the work of elimination, such as the kidneys and urinary organs, and the glands of the large intestines. In poisoning by alcohol, chloroform, hydrocyanic acid, opium, and the alkaloids, the local effects may be limited to the stomach and upper part of the intestines, but the three volatile poisons may be found in the serum of the brain. Lastly, animal or vegetable poisons taken in substance, whether as leaves, roots, fruit, or seeds, or as powder, may be found in any part of the alimentary canal.

Considerations such as these will determine the parts to be examined, as well as those to be reserved for further examination and analysis. In every case the whole length of the intestinal canal should be carefully inspected, and especially the gullet, stomach, and upper part of the small intestines, the cæcum and the rectum ; and these, with their contents (subject to exceptions arising out of the foregoing considerations) should be reserved. The examination on the spot must be so conducted as not to interfere with the more minute examination and chemical analysis afterwards to be made. The stomach should be first secured by ligatures at the lower end of the gullet and upper end of the duodenum, and then drawn out and placed in a large clean plate or chemical dish. It should then be slit from end to end in the line of the lesser curvature, its contents inspected and emptied into one of the jars, the inner surface carefully examined, and the ligatures removed. Double ligatures should then be applied to those points of the gullet and small intestines which present characteristic appearances. The stomach and the parts thus selected are then to be placed in one of the jars. The cæcum, with some inches of the lower part of the small and upper part of the large intestines, should be treated in the same way, as well as such other parts of the canal as are inflamed, or contain matters worth examining. In the case of the corrosive poisons and stronger irritants, the gullet, with the upper part of the windpipe and the tongue attached, will have to be removed and secured. Of the other viscera, the liver (or part of it), as the organ to which poisons are first carried by the circulation, the kidneys, as active organs of elimination, the contents of the urinary bladder, the heart, as a muscular structure rich in blood, and portions of blood itself, should be reserved; and in cases of poisoning by such volatile substances as alcohol, prussic acid, and chloroform, the serum of the brain and parts of the organ itself.

The organs and their contents, thus reserved for further examination, having been placed in separate jars, these must be securely closed by stopper or cork, covered with leather or stout paper firmly fastened round the neck, no sealing-wax, metal, or substance containing metal, being used. Tickets should then be attached, with numbers corresponding to those used in a description dictated at the time of the inspection, and verified immediately afterwards. The several jars should be carefully packed, and the parcel secured by seals. Letters of advice forwarded by post, and all other communications relating to medico-legal examinations in progress should be doubly secured, first by wafer or gum, and then by seal; and should, if possible, be posted by the writer; all other correspondence being carefully avoided.

That these minute precautions are not needless may be inferred from a fact reported by Tardieu and Roussin. Oxide and carbonate of copper were found on the mucous membrane of the stomach, through a large pin having fallen upon it after the autopsy.

In cases of exhumation, the character of the soil, the mode of interment, the state of the grave, of the coffin, and of the grave-clothes, as well as the position and appearance of the body itself, should be noted; and, if the earth is in contact with the corpse, a few pounds of it may have to be reserved for analysis. If the body has been interred in lead or a close-fitting coffin, and happens to adhere to its sides, the inspection should, if possible, be made without removing it.

The viscera and their contents having been carefully removed from the jars that contain them, and care being taken to preserve their identity, will have to be submitted to two successive examinations, the one physical, the other chemical.

1. **Physical examination.**—The physical examination will be directed mainly to the stomach and intestines, and the matters adhering to their inner surface. The odour of the contents of the stomach—as indicating the presence of alcohol, phosphorus, hydrocyanic acid, chloroform, and laudanum, and a few poisons less commonly employed—will have to be noted. If in doubt as to the existence of any characteristic odour, the organic matters may be warmed to a temperature not exceeding 100° Fahr. Each part of the intestinal canal should then be in turn spread out on a clean sheet of window-glass, with the internal surface outwards, which should then be searched by transmitted and reflected light, first with the naked eye, then with a hand-lens; its appearance described, and any substances that may attract notice by their form or colour particularly examined. Such small portions of the organ as present the most marked appearances may then be cut out, spread on clean glass slides, and examined under the microscope. By this means we may ascertain the kind of food that has been recently taken, whether it consisted of or comprised animal matters revealed by muscular fibres; or adipose tissue, with its polyhedric cells and fat globules wholly soluble in ether; or vegetable matters, with their spiral vessels, stomata of leaves, and chlorophyl soluble in alcohol, and imparting to it its own colour; sometimes also characteristic woody fibre. Or we may find evidence of a particular kind of farinaceous food in the characteristic starch granules of wheat, potato, rice, maize or Indian corn flour, oatmeal or arrowroot, or the spores of mushrooms.*

We may also find, more or less firmly attached to the mucous membrane, certain white powders, as magnesia or its carbonate; or the bicarbonate of sodium taken with a meal or after it; or calomel, taken as a medicine; or arsenious acid, given as a poison; and possibly undissolved corrosive sublimate, or imperfectly dissolved crystals, say of oxalic acid.

We may also recognise the corrosive action and characteristic discolorations of the mineral acids, and, when the stomach is far advanced in putrefaction, the sulphides of the metals (arsenic yellow, antimony orange, mercury black) or finely divided mercury

---

* For the characteristic forms referred to in the text, consult the "Micrographic Dictionary" of Griffith and Henfrey.

as a grey coating; as also the green aceto-arsenite of copper, the shining green and gold specks of cantharides, the brown powder of nux vomica, the blue of Battle's vermin-killer; and, as seen in the dark, the phosphorescent light of phosphorus.

The colour and consistence of the contents of the stomach will afford important indications; black, dark-brown, or greenish-brown grumous matter of the action of the mineral acids and oxalic acid on the blood, food, and tissues; and green matter, of the eating of leaves from the hedges. Sometimes, too, we may find fragments of leaves, buds, or berries, large enough for identification.

When the fruits of poisonous plants are eaten by children, we may find in the stomach or intestines the seeds which they contain. Those of the plants that require the microscope for their identification are shown in the annexed figure, in which—(1) Shows the seed

FIG. 58.

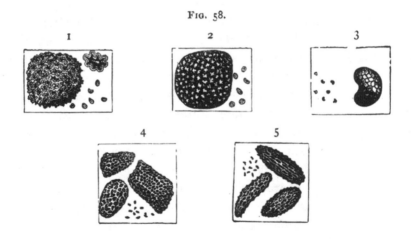

of Belladonna; (2) That of Hyoscyamus; (3) That of the Papaver somniferum; (4) That of Digitalis; and (5) That of the Lobelia inflata.

Portions of the larger poisonous seeds, such as stramonium, colchicum, aconite, castor, and croton, may also be identified by the colour and markings of their cuticles.

The advantage that may accrue from a thorough examination of the contents of the stomach is well shown by a case given by Tardieu. A child twelve years old died at school after ten hours of acute suffering on the day on which its stepmother brought it several good things to eat. Among the contents there were found certain fragments of crumb and crust of bread, which, when examined by the microscope, were found covered with fungous growth, showing that the bread was mouldy. Arsenious acid, in powder, was also found in large quantity. The fact of the mouldy bread was noted down, but no importance seemed to attach to it, till at the trial one of the witnesses, a servant of the stepmother, stated that her mistress was in the habit of carrying to the child slices of bread and jam, but that on the day of the death she said she would not take it, because the bread was mouldy. It had been in that state for one or two days.

2. **Chemical examination.**—Having indicated the precautions to be taken in searching the portions of the alimentary canal reserved, with their respective contents, for chemical examination, a few hints will now be offered under the distinct headings suggested by the following considerations.

The poisonous substances submitted to the chemist for examination may be in their pure unmixed form, whether solid or liquid, often in large quantities, or they may be small remnants of powder or crystal adhering to papers from which they were taken, or to cups or glasses out of which they were swallowed. In other instances the poison is dissolved in some common beverage, as beer, brandy, rum, tea, or coffee. In other cases, again, it has to be sought for in the urine ; or in the serum of a blistered surface, or of a serous sac after death, or, lastly, it may be contained in mixed articles of food of some consistence, spilled in the act of swallowing, voided during life from the stomach and bowels, or found in them after death ; or in such thick viscid matters as the blood ; or even in the solid structures of the body.

Systematic analysis. — Toxicological analysis presupposes a knowledge of ordinary chemical methods, so that it is unnecessary to describe them here. The toxicologist has usually to search for and detect poisonous substances in organic mixtures, and in the fluids and tissues of the body. Fortunately, in most cases, the symptoms during life, and the appearances after death, are such as to indicate the nature of the poison, and thus to make his research largely a question of verification ; but cases occur in which these indications are so uncertain as to necessitate an exhaustive examination for poisons in general. According to circumstances he may limit his research to the detection of a corrosive poison, such as a mineral or vegetable acid (especially oxalic) or caustic alkali ; of some volatile poison, such as phosphorus or prussic acid ; of some alkaloid or organic principle; or of some metallic poison. A research thus limited is comparatively simple. But where the indications are not sufficient to narrow the research in this manner, it is necessary that some plan should be followed in which the examination for one class of poisons shall not interfere with the analysis for another. Apart from the mineral acids and oxalic acid, the reactions and effects of which are usually so distinct as to require analysis merely for identification, the plan recommended by Otto[*] gives very satisfactory results. Search is to be made first for volatile poisons, next for alkaloids and organic principles, and lastly for metallic poisons.

In operating on substances involving important issues, it is advisable to use only one-third or one-half of the material at one time, in case of accidents, and to reserve the remainder for further research if necessary.

a. Search for volatile poisons.—Volatile poisons which indicate their presence by their characteristic odour in most cases, are to be separated by distillation, the phenomena and products of which give characteristic reactions. The chief poisons to be thus sought for are phosphorus, hydrocyanic acid, alcohol, ether, chloroform, nitro-benzol, and carbolic acid.

The substance is placed in a flask, acidulated if necessary with tartaric acid, heated in a water-bath, and the vapours condensed by a Liebig's condenser, and collected in the appropriate receiver. (See Fig. 66, p. 501.)

In order to insure the detection of phosphorus, the process of distillation must be carried on in the dark, to render evident the luminosity which is so characteristic of this substance. The special arrangements and mode of testing the distillate for the various volatile poisons will be described hereafter under their appropriate headings.

b. Search for alkaloids, glucosides, and other vegetable toxic principles.—Under this head is included the search not only for the alkaloids proper, but also for such active principles as digitalin, cantharidin, and picrotoxin.

Various methods have been suggested for the separation of these organic substances, but the method of Stas, as modified by Otto, and known as the Stas-Otto process, is the one most generally followed.

[*] "Ausmittelung der Gifte," 5te Auflage, 1876.

The method is based on the following properties of the alkaloids. Alkaloids are either liquid and volatile, as coniïne and nicotine ; or fixed, as strychnine, morphine, veratrine. Cantharidin and picrotoxin, neutral principles, and digitalin, a glucoside, are solid bodies.

They are all insoluble, or nearly insoluble, in water; but colchicine and picrotoxin are exceptions to this rule, colchicine being readily soluble in cold and picrotoxin in boiling water.

All the alkaloids are soluble in alcohol ; also in benzene, chloroform, amylic alcohol, &c. All the important alkaloids are soluble in ether, with the exception of morphine, which in its crystalline form is almost insoluble.

The salts of the alkaloids are mostly soluble in water, especially on heating. Some which are insoluble, or nearly so, are readily dissolved by the addition of a little acid. The solution of most turns the plane of polarised light to the left ; coniïne and a few others turn it to the right. Some have no effect on polarised light —e.g., veratrine and caffeine.

The caustic alkalies and the alkaline carbonates set free the alkaloids from their salts. When the liquid containing the alkaloid thus set free is shaken with ether or amylic alcohol, the alkaloid is dissolved, and remains on evaporation of the solvent.

The salts of the alkaloids, however, are as a rule not soluble in ether or amylic alcohol. Owing to this property, the alkaloids can be freed from organic matter soluble in these re-agents, and thus obtained in a state of purity.

The alkaloids, in addition to their special reactions, are, with few exceptions, precipitated by the following re-agents :—

1. A solution of iodine in iodide of potassium (Herapath, Wagner) —this gives reddish-brown precipitates.

2. Potassio-mercuric iodide—a solution of mercuric iodide in iodide of potassium (Winkler)—forming light-coloured precipitates, amorphous or crystalline.

3. Phospho-molybdic acid (De Vry, Sonnenschein). This may be made by adding to a solution of molybdate of ammonium, phosphate of sodium in the proportion of one-fifth of the molybdic acid, and sufficient nitric acid to make a yellow solution. This forms amorphous yellowish precipitates, some of which turn greenish or bluish afterwards. This re-agent also precipitates digitalin.

4. Phospho-tungstic acid (Scheibler)—solution of tungstate of sodium with the addition of phosphoric acid. This gives precipitates similar to those with phospho-molybdic acid, but less stable.

5. Phospho-antimonic acid (Schulze)—phosphate of sodium with the addition of perchloride of antimony. This gives amorphous whitish precipitates.

6. Potassio-bismuthic iodide—a solution of iodide of bismuth in iodide of potassium (Dragendorff). This re-agent gives amorphous orange-coloured precipitates. Among other precipitants are also to be mentioned picric acid, chloride of platinum, chloride of gold, perchloride of mercury, and solutions containing tannin.

Stas-Otto process.—The organic matters in the first instance, or the residue of the distillation for volatile poisons, are to be digested at a gentle heat for some hours with double the weight of strong alcohol, free from fusel oil, and rendered distinctly acid with tartaric acid. After cooling, the mixture is to be filtered, the residue washed with strong alcohol, and the mixed filtrates evaporated at a gentle heat in a water-bath to expel the alcohol. On the evaporation of the alcohol, fatty and resinous extracts separate themselves; and the watery residue is to be freed from these substances by filtration through a filter moistened with water. The filtrate is then to be evaporated in a water-bath to the consistence of a syrup. This is to be thoroughly extracted with absolute alcohol added in successive portions. The alcoholic solution is to be decanted clear, or passed through a filter moistened with alcohol, and again evaporated. The residue is to be dissolved in a little water. If the solution is very acid, it is to be cautiously neutralised with dilute caustic soda, so as, however, to leave it still distinctly acid, and then shaken up with ether.

Out of this *acid* solution ether dissolves, along with some colouring matters: cantharidin, colchicine, digitalin, and picrotoxin (also traces of atropine and veratrine). The ethereal layer, with these substances in solution, is to be separated from the watery layer, and the process repeated until the ether becomes no longer coloured.

On evaporation of the ethereal solution, cantharidin, colchicine, digitalin, and picrotoxin remain, along with fat and extractives. Hot water dissolves out colchicine, digitalin, and picrotoxin, but not cantharidin. The further characteristics of these substances will be found under their respective headings.

The acid watery solution which remains after the above extraction with ether contains all the other alkaloids. The ether is first to be driven off by heat, and then the solution is to be made strongly alkaline with caustic soda (or carbonate of sodium), and then repeatedly shaken with ether. Ether dissolves all the important alkaloids with the exception of morphine, which is to be extracted by the method given below.

A portion of the ethereal solution is to be evaporated at a gentle heat in a watch-glass, in order to ascertain whether any alkaloid is present, and whether this is liquid or fixed. The liquid alkaloids coniïne and nicotine remain on evaporation as oily drops of a characteristic odour. Should the presence of these be indicated, the mixed ethereal solutions are to be shaken with a few pieces of chloride of calcium in order to abstract the water and the whole evaporated in a watch-glass; fresh portions of the liquid being added successively until the whole of the ether is driven off. The residue is then ready to be tested by the general reagents for alkaloids, and by the special reactions characteristic of each.

If a fixed alkaloid is indicated by the preliminary evaporation, it will in general not be sufficiently pure for the application of the necessary tests. To effect this the ethereal residue is to be mixed with water and rendered distinctly acid by a little tartaric or sulphuric acid. The alkaloids are thus converted into acid salts, and are taken up by the water, while the organic matters are retained in solution by the ether.

The ether is to be separated, and fresh ether added if required to purify the watery solution of the salt still further. The watery solution freed from ether is then to be made strongly alkaline with caustic soda and again shaken up with ether, which dissolves the alkaloid again set free. On evaporation of the ether, the alkaloid is left. It may, if necessary, be again subjected to the like treatment if it is not sufficiently pure.

The residue is then to be tested by the general re-agents for alkaloids, and for this purpose the more or less impure and not distinctly crystalline residue which forms at the margin may be employed, while the more distinctly crystalline and purer material at the bottom is reserved for the special reactions of the individual alkaloids.

In applying these tests, a minute portion of the substance is to be removed and dissolved in a small quantity of water acidulated with hydrochloric acid. Drops of this solution may then be placed on slides, and tested carefully with the different re-agents. The tests may be applied on black paper to indicate cloudiness or precipitates, or on a white ground when colour reactions are involved and examined under the microscope when necessary.

In applying liquid reactions to such minute quantities, the following apparatus will be found very serviceable. The re-agent should be kept in a bottle furnished with a pipette, as indicated in the

FIG. 59.   FIG. 60.

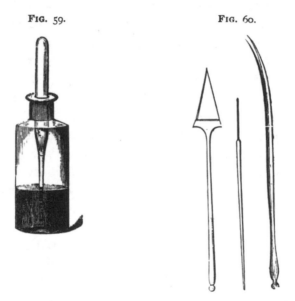

annexed figure (Fig. 59), and the testings, when carried on on a flat surface of porcelain or glass, should be made by the instruments shown in Fig. 60.

From the *alkaline* solution above described ether separates all the more important alkaloids, liquid and fixed, with the exception of morphine. These are the liquid and volatile alkaloids, coniïne, and nicotine ; the fixed alkaloids, aconitine, atropine, hyoscyamine, brucine, strychnine, veratrine, physostigmine, colchicine, and the glucoside digitalin ; and certain active principles which occur in opium along with morphine—viz., codeine, narcotine, papaverine, and thebaine.

It is necessary in this relation to remember that certain substances resembling in many respects the liquid and fixed alkaloids may be found in decomposing organic matter, and thus in the walls of the intestines and in the other abdominal viscera. These ptomaines or cadaveric alkaloids are separated by the Stas-Otto process. For an account of their properties and action, see under Diseased and Putrid Animal matter.

As has been stated, morphine is not (or only very sparingly) taken up by ether out of the alkaline solution. It is to be separated as follows :—The ether is to be driven off by evaporation, and the morphine, if present in quantity, can be separated in the crystalline form, by the addition of excess of a concentrated solution of ammonium chloride, and allowing the mixture to stand for some time. The ammonia takes the place of soda in the solution and precipitates the morphine in the pure crystalline form. If in less quantity, the alkaloid can be obtained better by shaking this liquid with amylic alcohol, which dissolves the morphine and leaves it on evaporation.

Or the original alkaline solution may be acidulated with hydrochloric acid, and then rendered alkaline by ammonia. The morphine is separated, and is to be dissolved out by shaking with amylic alcohol. If not sufficiently pure it may again be dissolved in acidulated water, shaken up with amylic alcohol, which will remove the organic matter, and then again rendered alkaline by ammonia and shaken up with amylic alcohol, as before. On evaporation of the amylic alcohol the morphine is left in a condition fit for the application of tests.*

After morphine, curarine and narceine may still have to be looked for, but they are not of much importance medico-legally.

Dr. Stevenson, in Watt's " Dictionary of Chemistry," 1890, suggests certain improvements in the process as follows :—The substance under examination is digested with twice its weight, or if a fluid, twice its volume of rectified spirit at a temperature of 35° C. After an interval of some hours the fluid is poured off, the solid matter being subject to pressure, fresh spirit subsequently being added, when it is allowed to digest as before. After decantation of the second extract, the process is repeated several times, spirit

---

* Erdman and Uslar employ amylic alcohol as the solvent, instead of ether, as in the Stas-Otto process, but though it is the best solvent for morphine, it has no advantage as regards the other alkaloids, and is, besides, extremely unpleasant to work with.

Rodgers and Girdwood prefer chloroform to ether as the solvent, especially when the presence of strychnine is indicated.

acidulated with acetic acid being added. The extracts obtained with the acidulated spirit are mixed together, but kept separate from those obtained by the use of spirit without acid, these being mixed together. The extracts are separately quickly raised to a temperature of 70° C., then each allowed to cool, filtered, and the residue on the filter washed with spirit. The extracts are then evaporated to a syrup at a temperature not more than 35° C., any excess of acid being neutralised with soda. The syrupy liquid thus obtained is drenched with 30 c.c. of absolute alcohol and well stirred. The alcohol is poured off and the process repeated with successive quantities of 15 c.c. of alcohol until it comes away colourless. The extracts are now filtered and evaporated to a syrup as before. The syrupy extracts from the acid and non-acid digestions are each diluted with a small quantity of water, filtered, and mixed together. They are then, whilst still acid, shaken with twice their volume of ether, the operation being continued until the ether, on the evaporation of a few drops, leaves no residue. The ethereal solutions are washed by vigorous shaking with 5 c.c. of water, to which a few drops of sulphuric acid have been added. The acid aqueous solution which was washed with the ether, and the water used to wash the ether after separation are mixed and alkalised with sodium carbonate and exhausted, first with a mixture of one volume of chloroform and three volumes of ether (previously well washed with water), and subsequently, two or three times more, with washed ether alone. The ethereal extracts are washed with 5 c.c. of water, then with 10 c.c. of water acidulated with H_2SO_4; and again with 5 c.c. of water alone. The acid liquid and the final wash water are washed once or twice with a little ether re-alkalised with sodium carbonate, and well extracted with washed chloroform and ether, and afterwards with ether alone. These ethereal extracts are washed with water barely alkaline, with carbonate of sodium, filtered through a dry filter, and evaporated in an oven under 35° C., in tared glass basins. When the evaporation is complete the basins should be dried at 100° C., cooled over sulphuric acid and weighed. To extract morphine, a well-washed mixture of equal volumes of acetic and ethylic ether is used.

The object of the repeated washings and transference of the alkaloid from water to ether and from ether to water is to get rid of fatty and other matters which otherwise would seriously interfere with the colour tests and also to enable a correct estimate to be obtained of the amount of alkaloid present. When the alkaloid is sufficiently freed from organic matter, the usual tests are applied to establish its identity.

Dragendorff's process.—This process is applicable to the separation of glucosides as well as alkoloids generally. In the following description all the bodies separated by it are mentioned, whether they possess a toxicological importance or not.

The substance to be analysed is finely divided and made markedly acid with dilute sulphuric acid. After dilution, so as to facilitate filtration, 5 to 10 cc. of dilute sulphuric acid (1 in 5) is added to each 100 cc. of the liquid, which is digested at 50° C. for a few hours, and then filtered. The residue is again treated with 100 cc. of water at 50° C., and after a few hours filtered. Both filtrates are mixed and evaporated to small bulk, after which the residue is treated with three or four times its volume of alcohol (90–95 per cent.), allowed to stand twenty-four hours, and then filtered. The alcohol is distilled off the filtrate, and the watery fluid diluted to 50 cc., and treated with petroleum-ether in the cold; this removes colouring matter, ethereal oils, carbolic acid, picric acid, and piperin.

The acid liquid may then be treated with benzine, which removes theine, cantharidin, santonin, cubebin, elaterin, digitalin, colchicine, absinthin, caryophyllin, cascarillin, populin, and traces of veratrine, delphinine, physostigmine, and berberine.

After the benzine treatment, chloroform may be used as a solvent; this dissolves especially theobromine, narceine, papaverine, cinchonine, jervine, picrotoxin, syringin, digitalin, helleborin, convallamarin, saponin, senegin, smilacin.

The chloroform is removed by petroleum-ether, and the acid liquid saturated with ammonia. From this ammoniacal liquid petroleum-ether removes strychnine, quinine, sabadilline, coniïne, and methyl-coniïne, brucine, veratrine, emetin, alkaloid from capsicum, sarracinin, lobelin, nicotine, sparteine, trimethylamine, anilin, volatile alkaloid of pimento. If the ammoniacal liquid be shaken up with benzine, the following alkaloids are separated:—Strychnine, methyl- and ethyl-strychnine, brucine, emetin, quinine, cinchonine, atropine, hyoscyamine, physostigmine, aconitine, the alkaloid of aconitum lycoctonum, aconellin, napelline, delphinine, veratrine, sebatrin, sabadilline, codeine, thebaine, narcotine. Extraction of the ammoniacal liquid with chloroform yields morphine, cinchonine, papaverine, narceine; with amyl-alcohol, morphine, solanin, and salicin, as well as the remains of the convallamarin, saponin, senegin, and narceine.

Lastly, when the watery fluid is mixed with powdered glass and dried, extraction with chloroform may yield curarine.

c. Search for metallic poisons.—The organic matters, or residue, of the operation for the detection of volatile and organic poisons, are to be finely divided and drenched with strong hydrochloric acid, and sufficiently diluted to form a gruelly mass. This is to be heated with the addition of chlorate of potassium in successive portions until the whole is converted into a yellowish liquid. By this method chlorine is set free and the organic matter destroyed, while the metals are dissolved in the acid liquid. (Silver, lead, and barium may remain undissolved.) The yellowish solution must be heated till all the chlorine is driven off.

The acid solution so obtained is to be filtered, and is now ready for the application of several preliminary tests.

To separate the metals, the liquid, properly diluted, is to be warmed, sulphuretted hydrogen led through it to complete saturation, and allowed to stand for many hours. From the acid solution sulphuretted hydrogen precipitates as sulphides, copper, lead, and mercury (dark), arsenic, antimony, and tin (yellowish). If no precipitate occurs, neutralisation with ammonia and the addition of sulphide of ammonium will precipitate metals belonging to the iron group—viz., iron (black), manganese (pink), zinc (white), and chromium (green). The material which remains after digestion with hydrochloric acid and chlorate of potassium may have to be examined for the presence of lead, silver, and barium.

Such is a general outline of systematic toxicological analysis, but such modifications as may be requisite in any given case must depend on the general chemical knowledge of the analyst.*

* In addition to works on chemical analysis in general, reference may be made to Bowman's " Med. Chemistry," edited by Bloxam ; Odling's " Course of Practical Chemistry " ; Horsley's "Toxicologist's Guide " ; Wormley's " Micro-Chemistry of Poisons " ; Winter Blyth's " Poisons, their Effects and Detection " ; Otto's " Ausmittelung der Gifte " ; Mohr's ",Chemische Toxicologie," and Dragendorff's " Gerichtl. Chem. Ermittelung von Giften."

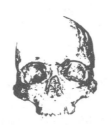

Other titles published by The History Press

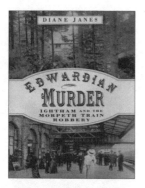

Edwardian Murder: Ightham and the Morpeth Train Robbery

Diane Janes

These two true crimes featured in Edwardian Murder bear all the hallmarks of traditional English period murder: steam trains, revolvers, an isolated summerhouse, retired army officers, parlour maids, to say nothing of conspiracy theories, murder, suicide, an execution and a love story.

978 0 7509 4780 0

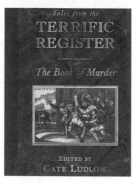

Tales from the Terrific Register: The Book of Murder

Edited by Cate Ludlow

This selection contains the most gruesome tales from this 185-year-old publication. Including 'the horrible murder of a child by starvation', dreadful executions, foul tortures and one of the earliest mentions of a now notorious killer who turned his victims into pies, it will chill all but the sturdiest of hearts.

978 0 7524 5266 1

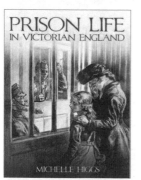

Prison Life in Victorian England

Michelle Higgs

Find out what life in prison was really like for the Victorian convict and prisoner, and also for the prison officers who looked after them. Using original prison records, contemporary sources and testimony from convicts, prisoners and prison officers, this book examines every aspect of the Victorian English prison to bring this fascinating period of social history to life.

978 0 7524 4255 6

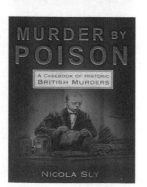

Murder by Poison

Nicola Sly

Along with the most notorious cases of murder by poison in the country, this book also features many of the cases that did not make national headlines, examining not only the methods and motives but also the real stories of the perpetrators and their victims.

978 0 7524 5065 0

Visit our website and discover thousands of other History Press books.

www.thehistorypress.co.uk

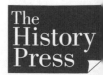